B&T
1-8-98
$11.95

BREAST CANCER

A HUSBAND'S STORY

by Bruce Sokol
with John Falkenberry

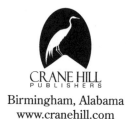

CRANE HILL
PUBLISHERS
Birmingham, Alabama
www.cranehill.com

© Copyright 1997 Bruce Sokol and John Falkenberry

All rights reserved
Printed in the United States of America
Published by Crane Hill Publishers, Birmingham, Alabama

Library of Congress Cataloging-in-Publication Data

Sokol, Bruce, 1944-
Breast cancer: a husband's story/by Bruce Sokol; with John
Falkenberry.
     p.   cm.
ISBN 1-57587-063-0
1. Sokol, Deidre Bergeron—Health. 2. Sokol, Bruce, 1944-   .
3. Breast—Cancer—Patients—United States—Biography.
4. Breast—Cancer—Patients—United States—Family
relationships. I. Falkenberry, John, 1943-   . II. Title.
RC280.B8S585   1997
362.1'9699449'0092—dc21
[B]   97-31026
                                           CIP

Dedication

D.D. and I are very fortunate to be surrounded by many wonderful friends and family members who helped us make it through this excruciating ordeal. In deep appreciation for your faithful caring, I dedicate this book to each of you.

—*Bruce Sokol*

For Ellen, may we come no closer to experiencing this hideous disease than through the words of this book; and for Bud.

—*John Falkenberry*

Table of Contents

About the Authors

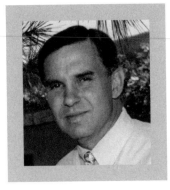

Bruce Sokol grew up in Birmingham, Alabama. After graduating from the University of Alabama in 1966, he served as an officer in the U.S. Army. Bruce currently works as financial consultant, and he plays an active role in a number of civic, religious, and business organizations. In 1995 he founded the Breast Cancer Research Foundation of Alabama.

Bruce lives in Birmingham with his wife, D.D., and their son Ben. He has three grown children, Adam, Jennifer, and Alex; a daughter-in-law, Caryn; and a granddaughter, Emily Hannah.

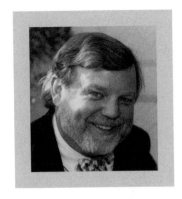

John Falkenberry, a native of Selma, Alabama, has practiced law in Birmingham for more than twenty-five years and is currently pursuing a career as a writer. Although *Breast Cancer: A Husband's Story* is his first book, John grew up in a newspaper family and for several years was a regular contributor to "Cordon Bleu and Barbecue," a weekly restaurant review column in *The Birmingham News*. He also enjoys acting and has appeared in more than twenty community theater productions.

John lives in Birmingham with his wife, Ellen, and their cats, Charlene, Edgar, and Boutros Boutros-Ghali.

Acknowledgments

Special thanks to my friend Melissa Springer, who planted the seed for this book and told me to speak from the heart and write with courage, truth, and honesty.

Special thanks also to the staff of Crane Hill Publishers for their help, encouragement, and support. I leaned heavily on them the whole way, and I suspect there were times they regretted taking on this project—but they never let me down.

Many thanks to all our doctors, nurses, and other health care professionals for getting us through the first inning of a game we intend to take into extra innings.

Many thanks also to the cancer researchers whose behind-the-scenes work provided the drugs and treatments that enabled us to win the first inning. We're counting on you to keep pressing on toward finding a cure so we can win the game.

And most importantly, thanks to D.D., who not only gave her okay but also put up with me throughout this project.

—*Bruce Sokol*

I am indebted to Bruce, my dear friend for more than thirty years, for inviting me into this endeavor, and to D.D. for her strength, courage, and honesty, all of which made this project a rewarding experience. I am most grateful to my parents, Roswell and Eleanor Falkenberry, for being both literate and literary and for exhorting me to be so. Many thanks to Ellen Sullivan and Crane Hill Publishers for their dedication to both breast cancer victims and their husbands, and for believing in this project. Kudos to our editor, Norma McKittrick, for her patience and perception. Thanks also to Dr. John Carpenter, for allowing me a small look into his world; to Arthur Capell, for teaching me to recognize the difference between horse sense and horsefeathers, and how to knock out copy on that old Underwood manual without really knowing how to type; and to many, many others, for encouragement and enthusiasm—you know who you are.

—John Falkenberry

Foreword

by John Falkenberry

In May 1995, a week or so before D.D. Sokol was diagnosed with breast cancer, I learned that I had prostate cancer. I was, in several ways, very lucky. Prostate cancer could be cured, and Dr. Jeffrey Cohn had every expectation that my surgery would, as he put it, "get you well again."

But having a serious disease, even one that could be remedied, certainly brought into focus what is and is not important in my life. I recalled the night my little brother told me that he had AIDS. After we'd cried for a while, Bud told me that having a terminal illness had at least one virtue—living life one day at a time had become much easier for him. I later saw that premise in the flesh. During his two-year fight with AIDS, Bud learned how to squeeze the very most out of every day as if each one was his last. As a result those years were, as strange as it may seem, the best of his life. While I knew I wasn't likely to die of prostate cancer, recalling Bud's words compelled me to take a very long, clear look at my own mortality. I was determined to live my life differently and, if I could, learn something of what he showed me.

The outlook is not as clear for D.D., and she and Bruce face a long, uphill climb. By the time Dr. Cohn had removed my cancerous prostate gland two days after the Fourth of July, D.D. was only about halfway through her first round of chemotherapy. By the time she had her mastectomy, two months later, I was on the road to recovery and feeling pretty well. I visited D.D. at the hospital shortly after her surgery and was astonished by her courageous, nearly intrepid attitude in the face of physical pain and a potentially fatal disease. I went home feeling even more fortunate. Everyone, including myself, had high hopes for D.D.'s full recovery, but we went on with our own lives too. My life as I then saw it did not include writing a book, certainly not a book about breast cancer.

A little more than a year later I decided to take a sabbatical from the practice of law, which had consumed me for more than twenty-five years. I was not exactly looking for a new career—I just wanted to think about my life and what other things I might like to try. The law had been good to me all right, but as with almost every one of my contemporaries, I was burned out and badly so. In the past when I had occasionally taken time off to try to regenerate my enthusiasm and dedication, I had found it harder and harder to come back to my practice. I needed to do something else, for a while at least. Maybe writing, I told myself.

And the opportunity was right in front of me, although I did not see it at first. My friend Melissa Springer, a fabulously talented photographer and equally fabulous person, had just completed a beautiful, powerful photo-essay book about breast cancer survivors, *A Tribe of Warrior Women*, which was published by Crane Hill Publishers. She recently had gotten to know Bruce and D.D. well enough to include a portrait of them in her book. (That photograph also appears on the cover of this book.) Bruce, who was the only husband included in *A Tribe of Warrior Women*, had become involved in the fight against breast cancer, and Melissa suggested that he write a book about it from a man's perspective. Other people involved with Melissa's book, including the Crane Hill folks, began encouraging the idea.

Bruce was intrigued by the idea, but he wasn't a writer. He would need someone to write his story, a coauthor. When Bruce casually mentioned the concept to me, I suddenly heard myself say to him, "Shoot, I could write it with you" or something equally profound. After all, who was better suited than a cancer survivor himself who also had first-hand knowledge of much of Bruce and D.D.'s story? I have known Bruce and D.D. for many years, have celebrated family occasions with them, had been with them at the hospital during D.D.'s surgery, and have supported them in their continuing battle with cancer. I had a wealth of research already in my head!

So our partnership began. With time on my hands and writing in my soul, I set about putting Bruce's story into words. Bruce recorded his thoughts on tape; I listened carefully, gently probed for more information when necessary, and then composed the sentences that form the small volume you now hold in your hands.

Living vicariously through the Sokols' ordeal was neither easy nor pleasant, even though I'd witnessed much of it firsthand. Breast cancer is a horrible disease that often bears grisly consequences for its victims. I want D.D. and Bruce's story to have a happy ending, and it may still have one. D.D is one remarkably strong woman, and if that counts for anything in this deadly game, she has a good chance of living a long time. I hope she does.

Birmingham, Alabama
July 1997

Introduction

by Bruce Sokol

One question I have been asked time and time again is why I would want to write a book that would expose the most private parts of D.D.'s and my physical and emotional lives. The fact is that in fighting breast cancer our lives have already been exposed to innumerable doctors, nurses, insurance people, family members, friends, and even strangers in waiting rooms. Quite frankly, there's not much left to hide.

I chose to write this book because when I needed practical help and advice in dealing with D.D.'s breast cancer, I couldn't find it. I found myself hung out there alone. All the focus, as it should be, was on the patient, my wife. I found more than enough books, magazines, and brochures about breast cancer, but nothing about how to help someone with breast cancer, how to be a strong caregiver, how to take care of yourself so you can be a strong caregiver. I want to share what I have learned so others will be better prepared than I was.

I am not looking for attention by telling my story, and I never dreamed that someday I would write a book—especially a book about fighting breast cancer. Although I have written this book to help others, in all honesty I have some underlying self-serving motives.

First, I hope that if this book helps even just one person, maybe something good will happen to D.D. and me. You see, I really believe that what goes around, comes around.

Second, since the day D.D. was diagnosed, hardly a minute has passed that I haven't thought about breast cancer. Writing this book has enabled me to put a positive spin on those thoughts, even though dredging up sad memories has been tougher than I expected. I kept taking encouragement from the hope that something good may come from this project.

Last, I will donate whatever proceeds I receive from the sale of this book to breast cancer research, the best way I know to fight this silent, vicious, bitter enemy that continues to threaten my wife. I am hopeful some new drug is in the works that will prolong the length and quality of her life, and I want to raise money for research now while D.D. is alive, while it can make the most difference for both of us.

Even though I had the firsthand experience of helping my wife fight cancer and was willing to share it, I needed a writer, someone who could take my myriad thoughts and form them into a book. I turned to my good friend John Falkenberry, one of the brightest, most dedicated people I know. John and I have been close friends since our University of Alabama days in the sixties, and he knows me through and through. Ironically John was diagnosed with prostate cancer shortly before D.D.'s diagnosis, and his own experience has enabled him to write about fighting cancer from the inside out. John made a complete recovery and took a sabbatical from his law practice about the time I was getting started on this project. Things just fell into place for him to collaborate with me. I couldn't have chosen a better coauthor.

Birmingham, Alabama
July 1997

BREAST CANCER

A HUSBAND'S STORY

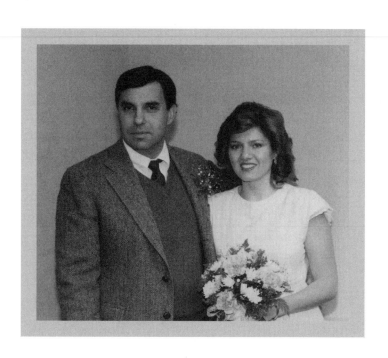

BASEBALL AND BAD NEWS

My youngest son, Ben Andrew Sokol, couldn't care less about baseball except as a social activity. He isn't a very good player either, but he enjoys being on the team because he likes being with his buddies. This has been more than a little disconcerting for me, a competitive guy who coached my other kids, worrying all along about their batting averages and won-lost records—as well as their fragile egos. So Ben's mother and I decided early on that I would never coach his teams, reasoning that both he and I would fare better with me just watching from the stands.

On Monday, May 8, 1995, though, I was pressed into service when one of Ben's regular coaches couldn't make the game. I was glad to help, but as the afternoon wore on, my thoughts drifted farther and farther away from young boys and baseball. It was pretty much a no-brainer—the teams used a pitching machine, so all the coaches really had to do was keep order. Besides, it was a day unlike any other I had ever known, and I had a lot more than baseball on my mind.

My wife and Ben's mother, Deidre Bergeron Sokol, who is "D.D." to everyone who knows her, had just returned from a long weekend at the beach with a group of girlfriends. I had not wanted D.D. to go on the trip because most of the other women were single, a fact that plainly and simply threatened me. But D.D. is a strong-headed woman with a mind of her own; she was determined to go on the trip, and she went. Her parents, Janel and Burleigh Bergeron, had come to Birmingham, Alabama, from their home in Lake

Charles, Louisiana, to help me take care of Ben. They had come along with Ben and me to the baseball game.

D.D. had a doctor's appointment and was planning to join us before the end of the game. Back in February she had noticed a tiny, pimple-like nodule beneath the nipple of her left breast. I felt the nodule, but as I told D.D., I wasn't a doctor—I didn't know if it was something to worry about or not. I asked her if it hurt, throbbed, felt hot—and she said no. D.D., who is a nurse, didn't believe there was much to it, and neither did I. I figured that if the nodule was cancerous, it would "scream out" in some way, and since it didn't, we decided to keep an eye on it and watch for any changes. D.D. began more rigorous self-examinations over the next several weeks but detected nothing different. More for our peace of mind than anything else, however, she scheduled what we both thought would be a routine mammogram for the afternoon of May 8th.

Her mammogram was scheduled for 4:30 p.m., which would give her plenty of time to get to the 5:30 p.m. game. As soon as the game began, though, I realized I was distracted—D.D. had never missed even one of Ben's games, and I caught myself time after time looking up into the stands for her. When it got to be six o'clock and then six-fifteen and D.D. still hadn't arrived, I became annoyed that she was late. Very quickly, however, I became frightened that something had gone wrong. My heart began to flutter and then pound like a drum as I searched my mind for a plausible explanation. Perhaps she had decided to stop by the grocery store or had gotten stuck in traffic. When she still had not arrived by the end of the game, my already queasy stomach was tied in knots.

Driving home I grew more and more jittery, and when I saw D.D.'s car in the garage but the house completely dark, my heart sank. I knew that the results of the mammogram could not be good. Janel must have sensed it too. She followed me as I hurried down the dark hallway and into our bedroom. We found D.D. lying on the bed in the dark, sobbing. The only words she could muster were, "I've got breast cancer."

An icy chill ran through my body as if someone had poured a bucketful of cold water over my head. I felt frightened, angry, and confused—all at the same time. As overwhelmed as I was, though, I realized that our lives were about to change drastically. What I couldn't begin to realize was just how drastic the change would be.

A cancerous growth doesn't always "scream out" cancer—it may not hurt, throb, feel hot, or give any indication that something is wrong. Cancer is a silent, vicious enemy that must be fought promptly and aggressively.

A CHAMP

As the notion that D.D. had cancer became less abstract and more real, the more angry I became. My first thoughts were, "Why her, why us?" D.D. was devastated of course, and neither of us could stop crying for very long. About all I could do that evening was hold D.D. close, cry with her, and talk a little. Neither of us slept a wink. It was the worst night I ever spent, a nightmare while fully awake. The night ended as the sun rose on that Tuesday morning, but the nightmare would continue with me for a long, long time.

D.D. tearfully told me of her visit to her gynecologist to review the mammogram results. She said that he seemed very matter of fact—even cold and uncaring—when he told her she had a lump that might be cancerous. He told D.D. he wanted her to consult with a particular general surgeon at the same hospital, a doctor with considerable experience in cancer surgery—it was just too much to deal with too soon.

Even though D.D. had known her gynecologist not only as a patient but also from her work at Brookwood Hospital, we thought it mind-boggling that he would simply ship her off to a surgeon, as if he wished to be done with her as quickly as possible. It sounded to me like business as usual, just another routine referral between doctors. We felt that rushing off to see a general surgeon was not the thing to do.

We were traumatized by the bad news but remained clear-headed enough to appreciate that while D.D. should not leap into surgery, it would probably be a waste of time to have a second mammogram. D.D. had looked at the X rays herself and, as an experienced nurse, could see that her breast was "engulfed with cancer," as she put it.

I blamed myself for letting D.D. go through the ordeal of the mammogram and talking with her gynecologist alone, but I soon realized that neither of us had expected anything other than normal results. I promised both D.D. and myself that she would not be alone during anything else she faced in her battle against breast cancer. We decided that she would not take her gynecologist's advice and consult with the general surgeon he had named—we would do something else, although right then we weren't sure what that something was. D.D. has not seen or talked with that gynecologist again.

After an hour or so of grieving heavily, we swung into action. We wanted to attack the cancer aggressively and started developing a plan. We called Mark Cohen, who is a gynecologist but too close a friend to both of us to be D.D.'s doctor, and asked him for referral advice. Mark recommended Dr. Marshall Urist, an oncological surgeon at the Comprehensive Cancer Center at the University of Alabama at Birmingham.

D.D. telephoned her sister, Tina, who lives in Houston, Texas, to tell her the news, and Tina insisted that we come out to Houston's M.D. Anderson Cancer Hospital. D.D. told Tina that if she had to be treated for cancer, she wanted to be at home, in Birmingham. That made sense to me.

The next day Tina talked with someone at M.D. Anderson who happened to know Dr. Urist and assured her that D.D. was in excellent hands. After Tina called and told D.D., we felt very comfortable about our choice. Little did we know that M.D. Anderson would play a significant part in our story later.

As I lay awake that first night, I thought back over the past few months. I knew D.D. occasionally did breast self-exams, but we never talked about them until the night she asked me to feel the small nodule that ironically turned out to be just the tip of a very big iceberg. I couldn't help telling myself that if she'd gone to the doctor right away, the cancer might not have had the chance to spread. By now we had waited two months to take the first step. Talk about uncertainty! There I was, second-guessing myself again. I didn't know whether D.D. would live or die, and I was already blaming myself for something over which I had no control.

The next morning D.D. told me that she wanted to do everything and anything she had to do to stay alive. I thought her attitude was incredible, but I had no idea what a physical and emotional ordeal we were facing. We agreed that we would not waste time feeling sorry for ourselves, but D.D. told me later that for a long time she couldn't keep from saying to herself, "Why me?"

While I believe that grieving is necessary and good, my philosophy is to get on with it as soon as possible. Neither D.D. nor I wanted to waste energy on things we could do nothing about—we wanted to direct all our efforts toward fighting the cancer. Now that we knew that we were dealing with the silent, vicious enemy of cancer and it had already taken a strong hold on D.D., we decided we would aggressively counterattack with everything we could.

I went to my office that morning, but I couldn't get any work done. Trancelike, I walked up and down the halls waiting to hear from D.D., who was calling Dr. Urist's office to try to get an appointment. D.D. is a tough cookie who can be absolutely single-minded and not take "no" for an answer, and she succeeded again—but it wasn't easy. Neither of us knew Dr. Urist or anyone on his staff, but D.D. was acquainted with a cardiologist at UAB whose wife was Dr. Urist's patient. D.D. got the name of the appointment nurse from the cardiologist's wife and called Dr. Urist's clinic. The appointment nurse told her that Dr. Urist was in the clinic that day, but the following day he would be leaving town for a week and already had a full schedule. By that time D.D. was becoming hysterical. Hardly able to say the words "breast cancer," she cried and pleaded with the nurse to let her see Dr. Urist that day—she could not wait another week. The nurse then contacted Dr. Urist, who agreed to work D.D. in that afternoon. When D.D. called and told me she had the appointment, I gave up on the workday and went home to be with her.

To say that the day was long and agonizing understates just how nightmarish the experience was. We arrived at UAB's Kirklin Clinic around noon, but we were not able to see Dr. Urist until 2:30 or 3 p.m. The wait seemed weeks long. We couldn't block out the zillions of thoughts blitzing through our heads: How bad is the cancer? What will they want to do? What can we do? Will D.D. die? The day became a replay of the previous night.

I wanted to be with D.D. through it all, and although I expected some resistance from the clinic staff, I didn't have to fight my way into the exam room or anywhere else. Wherever D.D. went, I went, with no questions asked. When Dr. Urist finally came into the exam room, he exuded confidence and warmth, two things we badly needed.

After looking over the radiology report D.D. had brought along, Dr. Urist said he wanted to perform a needle biopsy of the lump to make sure the mass was cancerous. In a needle biopsy, the surgeon aspirates the tumor with a fine needle and draws out some cells for evaluation. Dr. Urist was certain that the tumor was malignant, but the biopsy turned out to be negative. D.D. and I were incredulous—our emotions flip-flopped between hope and despair. "Oh shit," I thought to myself. "Is this what we're in for? How am I going to make it?"

Dr. Urist knew the mass was cancerous, but he was very cool and collected about the results of the first biopsy, never saying that the lab or anyone else had made a mistake. He simply said we needed to repeat the procedure, and this time the result was as expected.

The most frightening thing I saw that afternoon was the huge needle used for the biopsy. I never liked hospitals or doctor's offices, and this was no exception. I have a queasy stomach and abhor the sight of blood, but I was determined to be with D.D. through it all. Somehow I made it without puking my guts out right there on the clinic floor.

After the second needle biopsy was completed, we had a short wait before Dr. Urist came back into the room. Needless to say both D.D. and I were still scared to death. She was sitting on the exam table, wearing only a robe, while I was sitting in a chair across the room—neither of us said very much.

Dr. Urist came into the room, accompanied by his resident. Dr. Urist very gently removed D.D.'s robe to just below her shoulders, exposing her breasts. I had never experienced seeing another man touch my wife's breasts. But there I was and there he was, and I thought to myself that there was not a husband in the world comfortable with a male doctor examining his wife's female parts. Not only was I uncomfortable—I was also antsy and a little embarrassed. I sat silently and watched two men I did not know grope and gape at D.D.'s breasts. I kept telling myself that it was only clinical and that I wasn't bothered by it, but I was. You have to understand that before her surgery, D.D. had large, absolutely gorgeous breasts. Just the idea of these guys staring at them, doctors or not, drove me up the wall. Although there would be many other times and many other doctors who would touch D.D.'s breasts I don't think I ever really got used to it.

On one of those occasions, though, there was a bit of much-needed comic relief. Each time Dr. John Carpenter, the oncologist who tried hard to save D.D.'s cancerous breast, examined her he would put his face very close to her chest, almost touching her breasts. Once when his nose came particularly close, D.D. let out a nervous laugh. Then I laughed. It was just natural uneasiness, but Dr. Carpenter seemed embarrassed. Fortunately D.D smoothed things over by joking to him that because he got so close she could never come back to see him again. This time he laughed too.

Dr. Urist scheduled a series of tests to be conducted over the next forty-eight hours: blood tests, chest X rays, a bone scan, cardiac evaluations, and a core biopsy—in which larger sections of the tumor would be taken through a hollow needle. It was clear to me that Dr. Urist was looking to see if the cancer had spread. I was a nervous wreck; I could not eat or sleep. We called friends and family and told them what we'd learned, but that provided little relief. I was in another world, locked in a bad dream from which I couldn't wake. I couldn't seem to get anything right. For example, one morning when I made my regular stop to get a bagel and a newspaper, I put the receipt the clerk handed me into my pocket and threw the change into the trash!

I was very concerned about the tests D.D. was to undergo, but things were moving so fast that I didn't have time to feel sorry for either of us. There was the usual hassle at the hospital—filling out papers and answering the same questions over and over from department to department. Everywhere we went I asked the nurses and technicians whether I could be with D.D. during each procedure. Usually they let me go with her, although I was not permitted into the areas where they performed the bone scan and core biopsy.

D.D.'s attitude was great, much better than mine, and she actually helped keep me fairly calm, which enabled me to be a more supportive caretaker. Our positive attitudes fed off each other and kept both of us feeling upbeat.

D.D. was not only terrified about what was happening to her, but to make matters worse, she also was fearful that I'd do something to embarrass her, such as losing my cool and screaming at some blameless hospital employee—she knows me pretty well. Although I managed to stay calm and collected for the first part of each day at the hospital, by late afternoon I tended to become restless and frustrated. The days were very long, and waiting for test results was excruciating. I tried to understand the purpose of each test as well as what the results signified, but I did not always succeed.

The blood tests and X-ray results came back on Wednesday and were very favorable, but we had to wait until Thursday for the bone scan results. The doctors tried to be helpful, but they talked in medical lingo, so I tried to make some sense of their body language. I did not realize then that I should have asked a lot of questions. If I had it to do over again, I'd have written all my questions down when I thought of them and been sure to get answers—even though I might not like what I heard.

The last test of the second day was the core biopsy. I was not permitted to be in the room with D.D. for this procedure, so I tried to busy myself with other matters. I paced, read, telephoned my office, and made all the other calls I could think of—it helped to keep my mind occupied as well as pass the time.

When it had been much longer than the forty-five minutes we were told the procedure would take, I started going crazy with anxiety. D.D. knew me well enough to know what was going on with me, and after we had been separated for about an hour, she told one of the nurses, "You'd better go find my husband or he'll come back here looking through all these rooms trying to find me." I was about to do just that when the nurse came out and told me I could go in and see D.D. for a few minutes.

I will never forget following the nurse back to a small, dark room and finding D.D. stretched out on an exam table. Laying next to her was a very long, very bloody needle, and there was blood on the table as well. D.D. reassured me that she was not in severe pain and it looked worse than the procedure had actually been.

The procedure had been performed by a wonderful radiologist, Dr. Eva Rubin, and I thought I had seen her before either at the Jewish Community Center or my synagogue. She was not wearing the customary garb, and at first I didn't realize she was a doctor. She explained that she had inserted the needle into D.D.'s breast using a sonogram to find the tumors and cancerous lymph nodes. I learned that D.D. had multiple tumors, and I was able to see her cancer for the first time. My heart sank as I looked at the sonogram pictures.

I asked Dr. Rubin what seemed to be hundreds of questions: "Can her breast be saved?" "Are you sure the lymph nodes are cancerous?" "What happens next?" She was very patient and caring and transformed an utterly hideous experience into one that was not only tolerable but also educational.

D.D. and I saw Dr. Urist again the following day. He wanted us to consult with an oncologist, Dr. John Carpenter, who would be D.D.'s primary cancer doctor. I learned that oncologists administer chemotherapy and other systemic doctoring for breast cancer. Dr. Urist clarified that he was an oncological surgeon and that he would perform the mastectomy, if there was one—and he wouldn't operate until after D.D. first underwent extensive chemotherapy.

At first I couldn't understand it—if she had cancer, why not operate as soon as possible and cut out the tumor before it became more advanced? I later found out that D.D.'s doctors followed a technique developed by the French, and they would administer chemotherapy prior to surgery for two purposes. First, because chemotherapy sometimes reduces the size of a tumor significantly, it might become possible to do a less-invasive procedure, called a lumpectomy, and remove only the tumor and some surrounding tissue, rather than the entire breast. And by administering chemotherapy prior to surgery, the doctors could observe how the cancer responded to the drugs and how well the patient tolerated the procedure. Dr. Urist called Dr. Carpenter's office and arranged for us to see him the following day.

The oncology clinic was unlike any other doctors' office I had ever seen. It was a huge room, filled with maybe sixty or seventy patients, and many of them looked pale and sickly. Most of them had no hair; some were in wheelchairs or used walkers. D.D. was traumatized—as soon as she looked around, she began crying and hardly stopped for the next six hours. She told me later that her first reaction to herself was "Oh my God, I am going to die within six months!" My first thought was that it wasn't fair for my sweet D.D. to have to go through this. I also wondered whether she would live or not.

I recognized a fellow I knew casually. He was there with his wife for her chemotherapy. He recognized me too, and he and his wife came over and talked with us for nearly half an hour. They were very open and helpful. This was the first time either D.D. or I had spoken with another couple who shared our predicament. We mostly listened while they explained that the sessions passed quickly and weren't as unpleasant as many people feared. They said that chemo-therapy had taught them to be patient and set reasonable, attainable goals—in other words, we shouldn't bite off more than we could chew at the moment. They even assured us that their sex life hadn't been greatly affected. We felt better after talking with them, but we were still very fearful.

By 2:30 p.m. D.D. had completed her tests, but one of the results still was not available. The nurse told us to go to lunch and come back at 4 p.m. Already a bundle of nerves, I felt an almost indescribable fear. The image that came to my mind was of walking through a minefield—palms sweating, holding my breath, taking first one step and then another, never knowing when the next step would do us in. Then I started to get furious. We had been at the clinic all day and still had not seen Dr. Carpenter. Little did I know that this was a way of life in the chemotherapy department—just like being in the army, hurry up and wait for everything. Before we left, the nurse called again for the test results, which turned out to be nega-tive, so at least I was able to relax a little and eat something.

We came back at 4 p.m. and did not have to wait much longer to see the doctor. A small, amiable fellow, and very bright, John Carpenter was "just what the doctor ordered," so to speak. Friends had alerted us that his bedside manner wasn't the greatest but he was very good at what he did. However we didn't have any problems with his manner or with anything else about him. On the contrary—we felt very comfortable and confident with John Carpenter, and we would come to know him very well over the coming months. For the first time in days, I felt some relief from the mounting stress.

D.D. was still crying when Dr. Carpenter came into the room but calmed herself after we spoke with him for a few minutes. The first thing he did was give D.D. a complete physical. I watched as he put his hands all over her body, again telling myself that it didn't bother me—at least there was only one male doing it this time! Throughout his exam Dr. Carpenter spoke in medical terms. D.D. of course understood him, even though she was scared and crying. I didn't comprehend what he was saying, so I did not know whether it was good or bad. Not knowing what else to do, I sat there with my mouth closed, trying to pick up any nonverbal signals I could.

Dr. Carpenter recommended that D.D. begin treatment immediately with Adriamycin, which I later learned was among the most toxic of all the drugs used in chemotherapy. He gave the nurse a prescription and sent us off to the Infusion Clinic. The "infusion room," as it is called, is a plain, open area, perhaps fifty feet square and fitted out with a fleet of gray-vinyl recliner chairs, about ten against each wall. A nurses' "bullpen" dominated the center of the room. Televisions hanging from the ceiling blared away—soap operas, Headline News—it all sounded just like noise to me.

Admittedly neither D.D. nor I had contemplated such a sudden start to treatment. We had done nothing to learn about chemotherapy and had not even thought about the process until our consultation with Dr. Carpenter only minutes earlier. During that short time, however, I had painted in my mind a picture of a more personal and private venue. In fact it was one of the most depressing places I had ever seen. The room looked bleak and cold, and it felt grotesquely mysterious, although the recliner chairs reminded me of my days in my family's furniture business.

I wanted so much to be strong for D.D. and put on my best face, but I was actually sick to my stomach. At least the nurses were cheerful and friendly, which helped ease my nausea. Just when my stomach was settling down, it was time for D.D. to receive her first dose of Adriamycin, which is not only highly toxic but, I later found out, potentially cardio-toxic. D.D. risked serious side effects, including cardiac arrest. If I had known that when D.D. began her chemotherapy, I don't know whether I'd have tried to delay the infusion until we could study the options. What I did know was that the medicine injected into D.D. was a glowing, fiery, bright-red juice that looked like a concoction straight out of a science-fiction movie. That alone scared the hell out of me.

To no one's surprise, D.D. handled the treatment like a champ, with a smile on her face the whole time. She was always good about figuring out what she needed to do and how to get through a tough time, and she did it this time as well. It was hard for me to believe that within seventy-two hours after her diagnosis, she had already begun chemo-therapy. But we had decided to be as aggressive as possible in fighting the cancer, and I was relieved that we were already fighting back as fast and hard as we could.

The red solution they injected into her body looked as aggressive as it was supposed to be. D.D. received some strong antinausea medication, but she was prepared to be pretty sick for a few days. The nurses advised us that she would lose her hair in about two weeks, and on the way home we were laughing about how she was going to look with a bald head when we suddenly realized that my oldest son, Adam, was to be married in two weeks and two days.

Nothing in my life had prepared me—or could have prepared me—to deal with all of this.

> *Take some time to grieve and cope, but don't waste energy feeling sorry for yourself. Direct your energy toward fighting the cancer.*
>
> *Just physically being with your wife through the endless hours of tests and treatments will help her fight breast cancer.*
>
> *Keep a positive attitude—it will help both of you stay upbeat.*

BAGGAGE

I was born on July 4, 1944, and have always felt very fortunate to have grown up in a moderately affluent home and with a minimum of unpleasant experiences. As was the case for so many of us war babies, my parents were busy catching up with their lives and did not spend a lot of time with me. So I had to feel my way through childhood, make my own decisions, and develop most of my values on my own. My father, Max, seemed to work all the time in the family furniture business and was seldom at home. My mother, Sara, was a housewife who did her own thing, leaving my sister, brother, and me to make our own choices. For the most part I chose to do the things I thought would please my parents.

In the fifties the streets were safe, families left their homes unlocked, and television, still in its infancy, didn't have the powerful effect on young people that it does today. We all had a good time, and I don't remember having any of the fears that abound today. We didn't see pictures of carnage caused by storms, war, and crime. There was the polio epidemic, but it was trifling compared to the horror of AIDS. We had Chevy convertibles, sock hops, and drive-in movies; Ike was president, Elvis was on his way to becoming the King, and Bear Bryant heard Mama calling him home to coach the University of Alabama football team. It was a good time to be alive, and I took advantage of my good fortune.

Although I had some successes both during and after those early years, I have always thought of myself as an average person leading a traditional, largely undistinguished life. My few accomplishments hardly raised me above the crowd. I was always good at sports, and I became a proficient golfer and ran marathons. I was popular, made good grades in college, and was moderately successful in business. The driving force in my life was my desire to please those people I felt I needed to please—my parents, my wife, my children, my friends, even my pets. I always tried to do what everyone expected of me; I didn't want to disappoint anyone.

That's as true today as when I was growing up. I know I am misunderstood by people, even folks who know me well. My sense of humor is dry and sarcastic. I'm sure I offend many people, especially those who don't know me so well. What they don't know is that I care profoundly for other people and I have deep compassion and empathy for others. I often think back about how I got to this place in my life.

Following high school I enrolled at the University of Alabama, where I studied business and met Bobbi Silver. She was the perfect girl for me—and she fit right in with my life's plan to please everyone around me, especially my parents. We dated throughout college and were married shortly after our graduation.

Following my tour of duty in Okinawa with Uncle Sam, Bobbi and I resolutely set out to do all the right things—we came home from the army, I got a job, and we started having children. Our life together seemed to come right out of a fairy tale. We had three wonderful children, Adam, Jennifer, and Alex. I was successful enough in my business to allow us to build our dream house. We had good friends and a nice family. Despite all of this, however, we did not live happily ever after—our fairy tale ended in divorce in 1983. It's a sad ending that has left me with a sense of disappointment.

By the 1980s my life had changed significantly. Not only was I just going through the motions in my marriage, but I was also just going through the motions in the rest of my life. My family's furniture business continued to be moderately successful and I was active in my synagogue, the Jewish Community Center, and the University of Alabama's local alumni group. But I continued to feel average and ordinary; something was missing. I was completely dissatisfied with where I was in my life. Some people would call my situation a midlife crisis, but I never saw it like that. I simply wanted something more—or at least something different—out of life.

I decided to leave my family's furniture business. Although the business was still fairly successful, I was faced with having to move the store to a new location, and I just didn't have it in me to do that. I was at a crossroads and staring a career change square in the face. So as it turned out, in my mid-thirties I didn't just change careers, I changed almost everything in my life.

About this time I met Deidre "D.D." Bergeron, a young nurse from Lake Charles, Louisiana. D.D. had worked her way through McNeese State University School of Nursing and had recently moved to Birmingham. D.D. was unlike anyone I'd ever known. She was from a totally different ethnic background—she was Cajun and Catholic, and she was substantially younger than me, almost fifteen years. What struck me most about her was her genuineness—she was completely open and without pretense of any kind. I could see myself falling in love with her, but I couldn't see her falling in love with me. For some reason, though, she did. D.D. and I were married in 1986.

Although we had many good times in the first years of our marriage, there were many, many difficulties: D.D.'s adjustment to being a stepmother, my three children's adjustment to D.D., and Bobbi's residual angry feelings about our divorce. D.D.'s willingness to compromise and sacrifice got us through those tough years and strengthened our bond. Bobbi remarried several years ago to a wonderful fellow, Jim May. It surprised—and pleased—me that Bobbi was one of the first people to call D.D. after her diagnosis to say how sorry she was and to offer assistance. Strangely, D.D.'s breast cancer seems to have brought the two of them together as nothing else could, and Bobbi and her family have continued to be supportive.

After four years of marriage D.D. and I separated for several months, and at one point we were literally one car and a dining room table away from a divorce. Fortunately we made the decision to reconcile, and we did so with a stronger commitment to each other than when we first married. That commitment has been a big plus in our fight against cancer.

When D.D. was diagnosed I had only limited experience with cancer of any kind. When I was growing up, people didn't talk openly about cancer and the media did not have much to say about the disease either. Steve Mazer, a childhood friend, came down with Hodgkin's disease when we were fifteen or sixteen years old. A short, stocky kid who was very strong and a good athlete, Steve worked out with weights before he got sick and had great natural muscle tone. I remember visiting him right before he died, and I'll never forget just how frail he looked. He weighed only seventy-five pounds, maybe less.

There was cancer in my family too. My sister Sandra was diagnosed with thyroid cancer when she was in her early twenties. I knew that cancer was something extremely serious and was afraid that Sandra might die—and I was relieved when she didn't, but I didn't know any details about her treatment since my parents never talked about it. Like so many people of their generation, my parents tried to protect their children from painful situations and often withheld information from us.

They did the same thing when my maternal grandmother was diagnosed with breast cancer in the early 1960s. My parents did tell me that she was going to have one of her breasts removed, but not much more than that. I felt frightened for my grandmother, but I was more intrigued with the details of her surgery. Unfortunately for my curiosity, breast cancer was definitely not a disease anyone talked about. Although my grandmother lived almost another twenty years, I never really knew anything about her treatment.

I had a very close relationship with another family member who developed cancer, my mother's brother, Louis Rogoff. We often went fishing, and he let me operate the cash register at his store. A heavy smoker, Uncle Louie had lung cancer and lived only a year or two after his diagnosis. I remember visiting him—he seemed to be dissolving right in front of my eyes. He had been a big, strong, rawboned man, but by the time he died, he was emaciated. Again, though, I really didn't know much about his disease or treatment.

Within the last five years I have had several other second-hand experiences with cancer through friends and coworkers. I sat with my good friend Larry Baker and tried to keep his mind occupied when his wife, Mary, underwent cancer surgery. I was in the waiting room when the doctor came by to talk with Larry, and I knew from the look on the doctor's face that the news was very bad. Larry went off with the doctor and then returned to the waiting room, grief stricken. He said there was nothing the doctors could do—the cancer had spread too far. I felt glad to be there to support Larry in his despair, but down deep I wanted to be far away from that hospital. Mary died almost a year later, after a courageous fight. Larry went through periods of denial—he'd say Mary was doing OK and he was encouraged about her recovery. When he'd get on one of those emotional highs, I wanted to tell him that he needed to be realistic, but I couldn't do it.

Recently my coworker and friend Warren Merrin died of lung cancer. I had known Warren long before we worked together, but being in the same office brought us from being acquaintances to being buddies. Warren was an Alabama sports fanatic like I am, and he used to come into my office first thing every morning with his cup of coffee and we'd discuss the previous day's happenings. Just last July, Warren and I enjoyed spending a day together at the Olympic games in Atlanta. In September he was diagnosed, and two short months later he died. I had seen him every workday, and suddenly he was gone. Warren's death was poignant and difficult for me to handle.

I have also recently lost Ronnie Noojin, a friend since high school. While Warren lived only a few months after his diagnosis, Ronnie fought brain cancer bravely for a year or so. Even so, it seems he also was gone too quickly.

It was shortly before Mary Baker died that D.D. and I separated for a few months. I remember comparing my situation with Larry's at the time. Mary was going to die—she would be gone forever and Larry had no chance of getting her back. I was so much better off. D.D. was away, but at least I had a chance of getting her back. Our separation was difficult, but I never thought that I might one day face what Larry was facing.

Hopefully that day is still far away, but the doctors have told us that D.D.'s breast cancer will return. It's slow torture for me, but I cannot allow my fear of the future to spoil the good times D.D. and I can enjoy now. We have learned to make the most of every moment and not put off doing the things we want to do.

A strong commitment to each other will be a big plus in your fight against cancer.

Don't allow your fear of the future to spoil the good times you can enjoy now.

Don't put off doing the things you want to do. Pack as much as you can into every day, but don't make a big deal of it—make romantic dinners, nights out on the town, trips, and other special times together part of your "normal" routine.

Don't use breast cancer as an excuse to avoid "unpleasant" things, such as evening committee meetings, you normally would do.

SPREADING THE NEWS

It wasn't enough that we had to deal with the bad news ourselves—we also had to tell our family and friends. Fortunately D.D.'s parents were with us the afternoon D.D. had her mammogram and found out she had breast cancer. That was good for all of us since they could immediately share our grief. D.D. mustered the strength to telephone her sister, Tina, that night; I can't remember who told her brothers, Carl, Kirk, and Vince. D.D.'s parents and Tina have continued to give us tremendous support, telephoning and visiting regularly. Her brothers came to see us before her surgery but have not stayed in close touch. I sometimes wonder if it's because they are finding it hard to deal with her disease.

Passing along tragic news wasn't easy for me. I didn't worry so much about breaking the news to my father, sister, and brother, but I anguished over telling my kids—especially Ben. How does one tell a seven-year-old something as dreadful as the fact that his mother has breast cancer? Even though Ben was in the house with us that first tumultuous night, we were incapable of telling him.

I had an easy time speaking to my then eighty-six-year-old father, Max, who had already dealt with an abundance of bad news over the last few years. It seemed to me that he could handle anything. My mother, Sara, Max's wife of more than sixty years, had died only six months before D.D.'s diagnosis. Max's younger brother, Morris "Munny" Sokol, passed away six months after D.D.'s diagnosis. Both my mother and Uncle Munny suffered agonizing, painful deaths—Uncle Munny had Parkinson's disease; my mother had emphysema. The years before their deaths were long and tormenting, not only for them but for all of us, especially for Max, who was always there, emotionally and otherwise. I didn't think about it until D.D. got sick, but Max literally stayed at Sara's side constantly during her last illness—he never gave up the fight. I haven't imagined Max to be my role model for helping D.D. fight for her life, but hopefully some of his sensitivity, humanness, and dedication has rubbed off on me.

Max is a prince of a fellow. He's a rock-solid guy, guaranteed. I know he's my father and I'm prejudiced, but ask almost anyone who knows him and you'll get the same answer. Max is a thoughtful, gentle, private man who truly cares about people. He's just plain "Max" to us, never "father" or "daddy." And he's "Uncle Max" to many of my friends. Max worries about his family but keeps his anxiety to himself. He does not share his pain with everyone, and does not need to. Max has had a good life, very good up until the time my mother's emphysema became completely debilitating. Before telling him about D.D.'s cancer I knew that he would respond to me with understanding and kindness. I was certain I could count on him for whatever D.D. and I needed—I wouldn't need to ask for his support. Max has always been here for us, coming by the house with little gifts for D.D. and checking in to see if we need anything.

I knew my sister and brother would also give us enormous support. I'm ten years younger than Sandra and six years younger than Jimmy, but despite the age difference, we've rarely had a cross word among the three of us. When I told them, they could hardly believe what they heard and immediately offered to help in any way they could.

Sandra, who had experienced thyroid cancer when she was in her twenties, was able to see our situation through different eyes. She knew how it felt to be as frightened as we were immediately after D.D.'s diagnosis. She helped us find ways to relieve our fears, and even though she lived in Louisville at the time, she called daily to help us air our feelings during that difficult time. Sandra is not only as smart as hell, but she also understands how people feel—and she knows how to listen. I could not have made it without her.

My brother Jimmy and his significant other, Lydia Cheney, are crazy about both D.D. and our son, Ben, and they worry about D.D. constantly. Jimmy is my boss, and he made it easy for me to juggle my work schedule and spend more time with D.D. I mostly worked on my own, but Jimmy made it clear that I should not worry about the pressures of my job. I cannot say enough good things about Jimmy. He told me, essentially, "You take whatever time you need to deal with D.D.'s health problems—I understand. When you can work, come to work. But when you need to be with D.D., that is where you should be."

May 1995 was to be busy and exhilarating for all three of my oldest children, and I had been looking forward to that month like none before. My oldest son, Adam, was engaged to marry Caryn Butwin on the Saturday before Memorial Day in New Jersey. Besides Adam's wedding, we had two upcoming graduations—my daughter, Jenny, from the University of Alabama and my son Alex from Mountain Brook High School. D.D.'s medical crisis threatened to undermine the excitement of all these family celebrations.

When we telephoned Adam and Caryn and told them the news, they asked only if everything would be all right. We could not tell them what they wanted to hear, of course, but we assured them that we would not allow D.D.'s health to interfere with their wedding. We agreed that even if D.D.

could not make the trip, I would be there. I felt bad for them, especially for Adam. I am very proud of him. He was born when I was only twenty-five, too young and immature to be a father. I was not ready to make the kinds of compromises parenthood demands, but somehow we got through it. You might say we grew up together. I am very happy that Adam turned out to be a truly fine young man. I'm also proud of the way Adam and Caryn have continued to offer emotional support, even though they now live in New Jersey.

Jenny was planning to move to Washington, D.C., to begin work for the Arthur Andersen accounting firm. She had spent the previous summer in D.C. as an intern on the staff of United States Senator Howell Heflin, had fallen in love with the city, and landed herself an excellent job there. I was very proud of Jenny, too. Smart as a whip with a fine college record, she knew how to get things done. She was much better at it than I ever was. She knew what she wanted to do, set out to do it on her own, and succeeded.

D.D. and I did not want to rain on Jenny's parade, so we decided not to tell her until after graduation. Jenny's relationship with D.D. had been cordial, but never very close. When D.D. and I married, Jenny was living with her mother, and her feelings toward D.D. largely mirrored her mother's feelings. When I told Jenny about D.D.'s cancer, she said she was sorry they had not been better friends. Our ordeal with cancer has brought Jenny closer to D.D. They now speak regularly on the telephone, and Jenny has tried hard to be supportive, as difficult as it is from a distance.

Alex is as different from Jenny as June from January. He's a sweet, personable kid, and I love him very much. His relationship with D.D. has been very strong from the beginning of our marriage, although they seemed to be constantly at each other's throats once he elected to live with us after Bobbi remarried. D.D. thinks I allow Alex too much freedom and leverage, and he doesn't always agree with how she runs our household, but the two of them have developed a close relationship.

Alex was taking his final high school exams when we told him about D.D.'s cancer. He was also trying to decide where to go to college. He strongly preferred the University of Alabama, where many of his buddies would enroll, while D.D. and I thought the University of Colorado would be better for him. When she got sick, though, we decided that we wanted him to be closer to home so we could see him more regularly, which suited him fine.

Alex's response to our disclosure was to ask a ton of questions. He had lost two good friends in accidents during the previous two years and he wanted to learn as much as he could about D.D.'s prognosis. He was especially interested in D.D.'s proposed treatment and details of her chemotherapy, such as the likely side effects. Throughout our ordeal Alex has kept his spirits up, which has helped our whole family.

Telling our son, Ben, was the most difficult and delicate task of all. Both D.D. and I dreaded it because we did not know where to start or where to finish. D.D. was in no shape emotionally to even try—she told me that she simply could not say the words to him without falling to pieces. As it happened, the task of telling Ben started off on a pretty funny note. Some forty-eight hours after her mammogram, D.D. thought it was time to tell Ben, and I agreed.

D.D. asked me to bring Ben back to our bedroom. I assumed that D.D. had some preliminary statement to make, but as soon as we stepped inside the bedroom door, D.D. looked straight at me and said in a very firm voice, "Tell him!" I knew D.D. had a reticent streak that sometimes made it difficult for her to speak up, but she usually took the lead in dealing with Ben, even when I was to be the heavy. So what she did was both surprising and amusing to me, and I laughed out loud, which really broke the ice.

I was able to level with Ben, as I felt I had to. I think adults tend to forget that kids have an extraordinary ability to sense that something is not quite right. For this very reason, children deserve to be treated like adults when it comes to being honest and truthful. My philosophy is that everyone—including kids—needs to be told what's going on as directly and quickly as possible.

Ben is a savvy kid and would have seen through anything I told him that wasn't the truth. If I misled him now, how could I expect him to believe me about anything else later on, when words might be even more difficult? I told him that his mother was sick, that she had cancer, and that she was going to take some strong medicine to try to help her get better. I told him that her hair was going to fall out, that she might have a serious operation, and that she was going to feel really bad for a while. I told him that she might die, but it would not be any time soon.

Ben understood what was happening far better than I originally gave him credit. He actually asked a few questions, like whether D.D. had lung cancer. We didn't mention breast cancer but did tell him she had another kind of cancer. We talked about how Mommy was going to need his help around the house picking up his toys and clothes and that he should not give her a hard time when she asked him to do something for her. By the time Ben left our bedroom, D.D. had tears in her eyes. She said that she was glad I got through it because she could not have told him without breaking down—they were simply too close.

Ben has handled everything very well. Only once has he volunteered anything to me about cancer. I was watching a television movie about a child whose mother died of cancer. Ben was in and out of the room playing, and I didn't think he was paying much attention. Suddenly he walked in and said, "I hope my Mommy doesn't die of cancer." After this he seemed to cling to D.D. a little more than usual and had a few behavior problems at school. Fortunately these problems were short-lived and diminished in frequency as D.D.'s energy level returned and she was able to dote on him as she had done before her operation.

Tell everyone who needs to know—including your children—as honestly and quickly as possible.

Talk with your family and close friends about how you feel. Don't press them to talk, but make yourself available in the coming days so they can talk when they're ready.

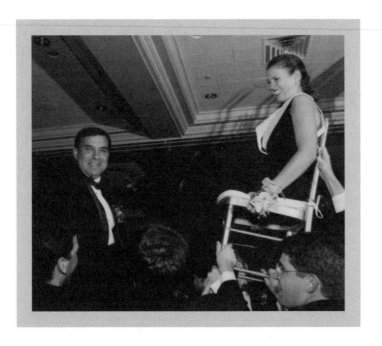

WE HAVE
BREAST CANCER

The first few days after D.D.'s initial chemotherapy became another of those "worst weeks of my life." I was far more anxious about everything than D.D. I felt very scared for D.D. and Ben—and for myself. I couldn't work, relax, eat, or sleep. Fortunately D.D. was able to sleep most of the time with the help of some strong antinausea medication, and when she was awake, she demonstrated a remarkable inner strength and fortitude.

D.D. was so positive. She threw all her energy into fighting the cancer, doing whatever it took to live, the side effects be damned. In my head I agreed with her that nausea, weakness, losing her hair, and maybe losing her breast— none of those things was an unreasonable price to pay if she could just survive. But my stomach was constantly tied in knots because I was not the one doing the fighting. While D.D. was engaged in battle with a killer, all I could do was sit on the sidelines and support her.

To help me feel that we were in the conflict together, even though only one of us could carry on the physical struggle, I started saying, "*We* have breast cancer." I used the catch-phrase "*We're* going to . . . " when referring to appointments, as in, "We're going to chemotherapy tomorrow."

Adam and Caryn's wedding was rapidly approaching and neither D.D. nor I wanted her health to steal any of the attention from their very special occasion. We considered not going to the wedding, but both of us had been looking forward to it for a long time. Not only would the wedding festivities be great fun, but we'd also planned a mini-vacation in New York City. We had begun to exercise more frequently, trying to get ourselves in really good shape so we wouldn't look like "beefy Bubba and his fleshy wife."

Fortunately D.D. decided she felt up to going ahead with our initial plans, and the decision provided some much-needed relief from our stress. Knowing D.D. would soon lose her hair, we went shopping for wigs. After trying on a few artificial tresses, D.D. said, "No way!" So we shopped for cute hats and caps instead and had great fun doing so. We bought so many that I teased D.D. that she had more hats than Imelda Marcos had shoes. D.D. was able to laugh about the whole thing—I think I may have smiled a little.

Although I was still scared to death about her health, D.D. made sure we departed for the wedding with a positive attitude. Once we arrived in New Jersey, we started having fun. We went jogging a couple of mornings and joined in all of the pre-wedding festivities. But on Saturday, the morning of the wedding, we were sitting around the hotel swimming pool when I noticed D.D. starting to cry. She was reading a book about breast cancer, and the negative statistics started getting to her. I told her to stop reading that book, and since then she has been more selective in choosing what to read.

At Jewish weddings the groomsmen take turns hoisting members of the wedding party in a chair held high above the heads of the other guests, bouncing and tossing each person in turn to the laughter and applause of all. D.D. felt good enough to take her turn in the "hot seat," and I felt so proud and happy to see her more like her old self. We all had a great time—even me. In fact, we couldn't have been happier!

D.D. looked absolutely radiant and was easily the most beautiful woman at the wedding. Sixteen days after her chemotherapy, D.D.'s hair was still gorgeous. Thinning a bit, but gorgeous nonetheless, thanks to the advice the nurses at the infusion clinic had given her on how to retard the loss of her hair. The nurses had told D.D. to put her hair up on her head and not to wash or brush it for a week prior to the wedding. She could clean her hair by dabbing it with a wet washcloth, but nothing more. And it worked wonderfully.

The following Monday, Memorial Day, we were in our hotel room in Manhattan, when D.D. awakened to find her hair coming out in large chunks. She asked me to find someone to cut her hair, but I had no luck since every shop in town was closed for the holiday. I was able to purchase some electric clippers at a nearby pharmacy, and the next thing I knew D.D. and I were in our hotel bathroom, shaving her head. It was an extraordinary experience, let me tell you. Not only were my hands trembling from fear, but the clippers felt very clumsy too. I tried to make jokes, but I don't remember if the jokes were funny or not. I do remember offering to shave my head too so I would know what it felt like and to be able to identify with D.D.'s emotions. She quickly replied, "Are you crazy? That would just call more attention to me!"

Because D.D.'s hair was so thick, the shears alone were ineffective. So I cut her hair with scissors for a while and then resorted to the clippers for a while, back and forth. The task took well over an hour. When the job was done, D.D. and I came out of the bathroom and joined Ben, Jenny, and a friend of Jenny's, who were watching television in our hotel room—and waiting anxiously to see what D.D. would look like.

For the first few seconds they just looked at her, but when D.D. smiled, they immediately smiled back. They just seemed to accept her changed look—which made it very comfortable for D.D. and everyone else.

D.D.'s bald head was very beautiful. I had not thought much about how she would look without hair, but I was pleasantly surprised and pleased with the outcome. Of course I was delighted with my barbering. Her hairless pate was perfectly smooth and glistened in the sunlight coming through the hotel window. Even without her hair, she was still a gorgeous woman. When we climbed into bed that night, I told D.D., "I never wondered about sleeping with a bald woman before, but I have to confess—I have had a secret desire to sleep with Telly Savalas!"

We were relieved to have the hair loss experience behind us, and with the tension broken, the rest of the trip was delightful. We took Ben to the Statue of Liberty and a couple of Broadway shows. He was thrilled by everything, and so were we. Because Jenny was willing to help us take care of Ben, D.D. and I had some time to ourselves and to visit with friends who had stayed on from the wedding. No one in our group of family and friends was the least bit self-conscious about D.D.'s baldness, least of all D.D., the woman of steel herself!

This happy interlude passed all too quickly, and we would soon be back home. Back into chemotherapy.

Even though only one of you is physically fighting cancer, start thinking and saying "We have breast cancer" and using the catchphrase "We're going to . . ."

Be selective in what you read about breast cancer. Chose books and articles that tell the truth about cancer but in a positive way; don't let negative statistics get you down.

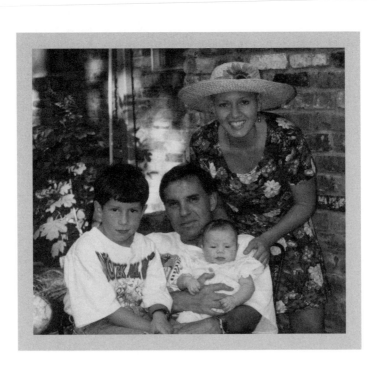

AREN'T YOU THE ONE WHO SAID YOU LOVE ME JUST THE WAY I AM?

When D.D. was diagnosed with cancer, I expected—and wanted—our doctors to operate and remove the cancerous tumor immediately. I didn't understand why she had to go through nine weeks of chemotherapy first, until Dr. Carpenter explained that he hoped the chemotherapy would shrink the tumor so they could do a lumpectomy rather than a mastectomy. From then on, even though I didn't want either of us to get our hopes up too high, I couldn't help holding onto the possibility that D.D.'s breast wouldn't have to be removed. It was a long shot, but it helped us get through the depressing weeks of chemotherapy.

D.D. handled the chemotherapy sessions courageously and remained in good spirits, despite the nausea and listlessness that accompanied each infusion of Adriamycin. The summer became a recurring cycle of treatment followed by rest and then more treatment. D.D. rebounded from each of the sessions pretty quickly and within a few days was able to resume her daily routine—aerobic exercise classes, yard work, even jogging. We made love frequently—we did everything and anything to try to make our daily life seem normal, whatever "normal" was.

Unfortunately D.D.'s cancer was aggressive and Adriamycin failed to shrink her tumor, which was large—about 7.5 centimeters in diameter. Dr. Carpenter decided to try Paclitaxel (TAXOL), a new, very potent chemotherapy drug only recently approved for the treatment of breast cancer. I was sorely disappointed that Adriamycin had not been effective, and although I had hopes that TAXOL would work for her, I wasn't sure I could handle the additional stress of trudging down to the infusion clinic for more chemotherapy sessions. D.D. remained upbeat, however, and her spirit lifted me out of my misery. I reminded myself that *we* had breast cancer and of course we would go back to the infusion clinic as many times as necessary. We would do anything and everything to beat *our* cancer.

Fortunately D.D. bounced back from the infusions of TAXOL as well as she had from Adriamycin. Even better, her tumor responded to TAXOL and began to shrink. We kept our fingers crossed.

The hope of saving D.D.'s breast ended, though, after three infusions of TAXOL—her tumor had shrunk, but not nearly enough to avoid major surgery. When Dr. Carpenter uttered "mastectomy," I knew I was not prepared to face having D.D. lose her breast. All along I had lulled myself into believing that somehow, some way, she'd get better without major surgery. But here we were, facing a dangerous operation that, under the best of circumstances, would change D.D.'s body and our lives forever.

Once again I felt frightened, angry, and resentful. I couldn't keep myself from comparing my mother's emphysema with D.D.'s cancer. Sara had contributed greatly to her disease by many years of heavy smoking. D.D. had done nothing to bring on her cancer—in fact, she was physically and spiritually strong and had done everything right to stay healthy. She worked out regularly, didn't smoke or use drugs, drank alcohol only occasionally, and ate healthy foods. Ironically, two days before she went for the mammogram in May, she ran for a solid hour and a half, longer than she had ever run in her life. The only thing that made D.D. a candidate for breast cancer was that she was a woman.

I thought it grossly unfair that D.D.'s beauty would be marred in the prime of her life! What makes breast cancer so abominable is that it attacks a very visible part of a woman's body, a part that unfortunately has come to symbolize the essence of femininity.

I knew that D.D.'s mastectomy would leave emotional as well as physical scars. Through it all, though, right up to the day of her surgery, D.D. rarely complained or felt sorry for herself—which helped me stay on a relatively even emotional keel. She kept that great smile on her face even when it would have been much easier to frown. She looked and acted more normal than I could ever have imagined. Sometimes I'd have to pinch myself to remember that she was sick. Once again, every positive thought that either of us could muster helped the other stay upbeat.

We scheduled D.D.'s surgery for Labor Day, the first date both of our surgeons were available. Dr. Marshall Urist would perform the three-hour mastectomy, and Dr. Jim Grotting would do the seven-hour breast reconstruction. Once the date was set, I had little or no interest in anything other than D.D.'s health—not golf, not work, nothing. D.D. and I spent most of the days before Labor Day together.

Still feeling afraid and angry, I decided that the best thing was to share my anguish with D.D. We had not talked very much about how we felt about her disease since the night after her diagnosis. Of course we had talked over her test results and chemotherapy results, but we did not dwell on the possibility of her dying anytime soon. Couples don't talk about the possibility of one of them being killed in a car accident, so why death by cancer? I also thought we didn't need to talk very much because D.D. kept giving me so much strength, which also seemed to help keep her strong.

D.D told me that she felt I was the one who had been strong, but I continued to worry, actually to obsess, about all the unknowns of her upcoming ten-hour operation: Could D.D. tolerate being under anesthesia for that long? How would she look after the surgery? How long would her physical recovery take? Would she recover?

For the first time I wondered how D.D. would react emotionally to losing her breast. We had so riveted our attention on the physical aspect of her treatment, that we had completely neglected the emotional. In a way that was good because I would have had a more difficult time handling the emotional aspect before. It was hard enough when I finally got around to it.

I was a total wreck by Labor Day—the dreaded day of living hell. I was more anxious and apprehensive than I had ever been before. That says a lot since I have lived my entire life with the *shpilkes*, which is Yiddish for "a bad case of the jitters." In the twenty-four hours preceding D.D.'s surgery, my nerves were completely shot. I couldn't eat. I couldn't sit still, but I couldn't make myself exercise either. I couldn't sleep, and in desperation I took a sleeping pill. We spent the night before the operation at home and arrived at the hospital's admitting desk by 6:15 a.m.

D.D.'s parents and her sister, Tina, had arrived in town several days before the scheduled surgery. Tina went with D.D. and me to the hospital, while Janel and Burleigh stayed at our house with Ben and Tina's five-month-old daughter, D.D.'s namesake.

When we checked in, D.D. obtained a copy of her hospital orders, routine records describing the surgery she would undergo. After looking at the sheet, D.D. showed it to me. Neither of us could believe that the hospital orders stated the mastectomy was to be performed on her *right* breast—the tumor was in her *left* breast!

I snarled, "How can such a prominent hospital make such an asinine mistake?" D.D. was not as perturbed as I was because she knew Dr. Grotting would be coming by before the surgery to make some marks on her cancerous breast to guide him in his reconstruction. She was confident that he'd get it right, and he did. I was already about to burst with anxiety, though, and what I saw as the hospital's inexcusable stupidity was just about the last straw.

D.D. left her room for the operation about 7 a.m. She was actually glowing when the orderlies rolled her gurney out into the hallway. I kissed her good-bye, knowing that the next time I saw her, she'd not be the same—her body would have been carved, sliced, and stitched. I kept telling myself that I wouldn't care how she looked as long as she came back to me alive and cancer free. I felt at peace with the idea that her body would look and feel different than before.

What I realized on the day of her mastectomy was that I loved D.D. more than ever before. I was afraid to love her so much, though, because I feared that my pain would be so much greater if she died.

As she was being wheeled out of the room, D.D. told me not to worry. Tina followed the gurney down the hall, and I think she would have gone into the operating room if the hospital staff had not turned her back. When Tina returned to the room, she handed me an envelope addressed to me in D.D.'s handwriting. In the emotion of the moment, I put the envelope aside—I couldn't bear to open it just then. I paced back and forth in front of the window for a long time, looking out and thinking how beautiful the day was—and that I could be playing golf and eating barbecue as I did on most summer holidays.

About 10:30 a nurse called to say that the first part of the surgery was over—Dr. Urist had removed the cancerous tumors and lymph nodes, and D.D. was doing okay. Dr. Grotting was about to begin constructing a replacement breast.

I remembered the envelope from D.D. that I had put aside unopened. I lay down on her hospital bed and opened it. Inside was a card with a cartoon cat sitting on a stool, deep in thought and with a faraway look saying, "I'm hopeless. I admit it." The message continued inside, "But aren't you the one who said you love me just the way I am?" D.D. had also written me a note that was as simple and beautiful as it was powerful.

Dear Bruce,

You are sitting in my room, and I am, well, you know where. I'm sure it's the middle of the afternoon. You are a runaway train, and I am doing great! Don't worry, this will be over soon and I will be back in my room. Please don't kill Tina! She is my only sister.

I can't tell you how great you have been through our ordeal. You tell me every day how much you love me, more each day, and I know the feeling. Every day my love for you grows and grows. This has brought us closer than I could have imagined.

So sit tight, try to relax, and I will be back shortly. We can start over again and have a wonderful life together.

I love you,

D.D.

Tears welled up in my eyes. How could D.D. be so strong? She was worrying about me! How fortunate I was to have her—I didn't want to lose her. I stared at the ceiling and let my thoughts wander for a long time. I even missed lunch.

Family and friends stopped by to lend their support and help me pass the time. I hadn't been keen on the idea of having visitors, imagining that it would be a major-league pain in the ass to entertain anyone when I was feeling so emotional, but my father, Max, and my brother and sister, and the others who came really helped me a lot. They brought food, books, newspapers, and magazines. I felt deeply touched, even though I remained in a fog.

At 1:30 p.m. the nurse called to tell me that D.D. was hanging in there with only an hour or two to go. I realized that Dr. Grotting was ahead of schedule, which hopefully meant the reconstruction was going well. Thank goodness the surgery would soon be over—I felt like I had been in the hospital room for a month.

Dr. Urist stopped by to tell me that his part of the operation had gone very well but he wouldn't really know anything until he studied the pathology report, which was due at 3 p.m. the next day. As he was leaving, the nurse called again to tell me they were closing the incisions. The operation had lasted between seven and eight hours rather than the expected ten. Thank God for that. Shortly after the nurse's phone call, Dr. Grotting came to the room and told me that he was pleased with the reconstructive surgery, the first of several surgical procedures it would take to create D.D.'s new breast.

D.D. finally came back to the room about 4 p.m. She had six tubes sticking out of her body—all of them filled with bloody, pus-like fluids. As happy as I was to see D.D., I didn't like looking at those tubes or the fifteen-inch-long white Hickman catheter that protruded from her chest. We had decided to have the catheter inserted so post-op chemotherapy could be administered through it and blood could be drawn out of it rather than having needles repeatedly inserted into her veins.

D.D.'s beautiful body had been hacked up even worse than I'd expected, but she was alive and the scars would heal. I was eager to see what her reconstructed breast looked like—I could not imagine how doctors worked such miracles.

I wanted to stay at the hospital with D.D. all night, but when Tina, who is a nurse, insisted that she be the one to stay, I decided not to make it an issue. Tina and I negotiated an arrangement—I would stay at the hospital during the day and Tina would stay overnight.

I went home about 9 p.m., hungry and exhausted. I ate a little, made a few telephone calls, and got ready for bed. As I crawled under the sheets, I took another look at the card and note D.D. had given me. I cried a little, took a sleeping pill, and was out like a light.

It doesn't matter whether your wife lives a healthy lifestyle and has no family history of cancer—just the fact that she's a woman means that she's a candidate for breast cancer.

Sharing every positive thought you can muster will help both of you keep your spirits up.

Your wife's body may be hacked up terribly during surgical procedures, but the scars will heal—the most important thing is that she's still alive.

Make love frequently—it will bring you closer together.

COMMUNICATING WITH EACH OTHER

Even though D.D. was home from the hospital and recovering steadily from her mastectomy and initial reconstruction surgery, it did not mean that the end to her treatment was in sight. We still faced months of chemotherapy—three more rounds of TAXOL followed by six infusions of CMF, a combination of Cytoxan, methotrexate, and FU-5 (fluorouracil).

Oncologists have prescribed CMF as "adjuvant" therapy when microscopic, undetectable amounts of cancer may remain in the bloodstream. Approximately forty percent of women who have mastectomies experience recurrent breast cancer. Adjuvant treatment increases the survival rate fifteen to twenty percent for those women. Since doctors cannot identify the forty percent of women who need this adjuvant therapy, a good number of women who have mastectomies get zapped with CMF or a similar combination of drugs.

D.D.'s post-surgery chemotherapy was somewhat easier because of the Hickman catheter we decided to have the doctors implant in her chest during her operation. We knew that chemotherapy can be very hard on veins and the catheter would provide a stable, portal for the IV needle, eliminating the need to find a fresh vein for each infusion. At first the catheter felt cumbersome and looked unattractive, but we soon became used to it and wound up laughing about it. I used to joke with D.D. that I was afraid I might get tangled up in it and accidentally pull it out, but it didn't get in the way, even when we made love. In the long run the convenience, comfort, and other benefits of the catheter far outweighed the few negatives.

Even though D.D.'s post-surgery chemotherapy was a little less arduous than the earlier sessions, it was another difficult experience for us. D.D. told me, "I'm sick of all this happening to me!"

Despite the stress of her treatments, our relationship seemed closer than ever. Before D.D.'s diagnosis, we didn't always communicate with each other very well. Both of us tended to hold our emotions inside, saying almost nothing about how we felt until one or the other of us would burst out in anger, often about something relatively inane.

As we worked together in our fight against breast cancer, we argued less often and with less intensity. We laughed off situations that formerly would have resulted in conflict. Don't ask me how we did it—it just happened, without a great deal of conscious effort. Because the serious subject of breast cancer and its treatment so dominated our conscious minds, we had little time for petty hostilities, and we naturally began to treat each other with more love and respect.

We have plenty to talk about—the details of D.D.'s treatment, her doctors, the infusion clinic, her exercise program, problems with the insurance carrier, and the difficulty of getting through her surgery. But we talk only indirectly about the disease itself and its long-range ramifications for her and us. I intentionally avoid talking about these morbid topics because I don't want to crush D.D.'s positive attitude. We just talk in general about the inevitability of death and my wanting her to stay around as long as possible. We still haven't talked about D.D. dying from breast cancer, although we both believe that cancer likely will shorten her life.

Fortunately I haven't had to deal with the untimely death of a family member. While I accept death as a natural part of life, I think that when someone dies young or unexpectedly, it's a tragedy—I feel like they've been short-changed. On the other hand, if someone lives a full life, their death can be a celebration of their life. I know that nobody lives forever, and my biggest fear of all is not that D.D. will die—but watching her die. I hope that when her time comes, she will die with dignity and very little suffering.

We wonder whether D.D. will be around to enjoy my retirement years with me. We speculate about how many more trips we will be able to take together, but not how many years she has to live. We watch virtually every television program dealing with breast cancer. We talk about new treatments and breakthroughs and how other people deal with the disease. Because we may have a limited amount of time left together, we want to live our lives to the fullest. There will be time to talk about death; for the present, however, we choose to focus on the positive.

I have carefully avoided engaging in dialogue about subjects that I consider uncomfortable and unpleasant because my philosophy has always been to keep as even a keel as possible by avoiding highs and lows. As Mel Brooks once said, "Expect the worst; hope for the best" or something like that. If you don't allow your expectations to go sky high, you won't be disappointed, and if something bad happens, you're ready for it.

I try to stay balanced by keeping my expectations realistic—it's something I've always done, but I never thought about it before D.D.'s illness. I believe that it's especially important in a time of crisis not to exaggerate feelings of euphoria or depression—swinging back and forth between these extremes can be emotionally damaging. When we received test results that were favorable, I would remind myself that winning one skirmish against breast cancer was not the same as just getting over the flu. On the other hand, when the test results were not in our favor, I would tell myself that it was not the end of the world—it was just a setback.

Although I try to avoid uncomfortable, unpleasant subjects, I have learned to start asking the doctors more questions. D.D. does a great job of this, often taking along a detailed list of questions and asking them over and over until she gets an answer. At first I asked questions, but then I got to thinking that perhaps there were questions I should not ask and information I should not know. I want to get inside the doctors' heads and find out what they really think D.D.'s future holds, but I am afraid to form my thoughts into specific questions. I'm afraid they will tell me something I don't want to hear, and with breast cancer more often than not they're just guessing anyway.

In the months since D.D.'s diagnosis, I've had many conversations with people who, with the best of intentions, told me what they thought I wanted to hear. Those people wanted to ease my pain by telling me that everything would be all right—which is not what I wanted to hear at all. I must have said that same thing to other people many times over the years, and it never bothered me until I was on the listening end of things. People want to make things all right, but they can't. What I wish people would say instead is, "I'm sorry to hear your bad news. I'll be thinking about you and D.D."

I most appreciate the response that came separately from two of my oldest friends when I called to tell them about D.D.'s breast cancer. Both David and John said something like, "Oh shit, Bruce. God, I am sorry." Nothing more. That did the trick for me—they said all that I wanted and needed to hear.

Don't hold in your emotions. If you need to cry, do it. If you can't bear for anybody to see you cry, find a place where you can let the tears flow in private.

Talk about anything and everything.

Don't waste time being angry at each other or anyone else. Keep in mind how small daily frustrations are in relation to the amount of time you still have together.

Try to stay on as even a keel as possible by keeping your expectations reasonable and not exaggerating feelings of euphoria or depression.

OH, MY
ACHING BACK!

We went to D.D.'s final chemotherapy in January 1996, nine long months after the first session. D.D.'s catheter was removed a month later, and the seemingly endless hours at the infusion clinic were over. While going through chemotherapy, we couldn't wait for it to be over. Once it actually was over, we felt elated and at the same time singularly insecure. I told D.D., "You know, I thought I'd be happy when this moment came, but it scares me that we're on our own." We had come to rely on Kirklin Clinic's now-familiar environment and staff members as a buffer between us and the great unknown.

After the last chemotherapy session, D.D. began taking tamoxifen (trade name Nolvadex), which has been used for the past ten years in hormone therapy for breast cancer survivors. Tamoxifen helps prevent the recurrence of cancer by inhibiting the effects of estrogen, a hormone that enhances the growth of malignant cells. Tamoxifen has minimal toxicity and the only major concern is an increased risk of endometrial (uterine) cancer. Tamoxifen has none of the usual side effects of other drugs, but because it inhibits the effects of estrogen, many premenopausal women who take it experience early onset of menopause or at least menopausal symptoms.

D.D. has experienced menopausal symptoms, but it has been worth it—tamoxifen has effectively reduced D.D.'s metastatic cancer into remission, which has given both of us renewed hope. What concerns us is how long the beneficial effects of tamoxifen will last. Dr. Carpenter has told us that tamoxifen is not effective for everyone, but if it is effective, its beneficial properties should last for five years. I've already started to worry about whether some new drug will come along in time to keep D.D.'s cancer from recurring beyond the five years.

With spring coming on and no more side effects from chemotherapy to slow her down, D.D. threw herself into getting back into tip-top shape. In addition to running the household, she worked in our yard—always a labor of love for her—she worked out, jogged, played with Ben, and generally stayed active. She felt pretty good, and I could see both her strength and her stamina on the increase. Her enthusiasm and energy were boundless and she tended to overestimate her physical capabilities, but she refused to concede any infirmity. For example, we were jogging one afternoon when she tripped and fell, scraping her hands and knees on the asphalt roadway. She was hurt and angry, but she got right up, blood dripping down from one knee, and finished the run without a word of complaint.

One of D.D.'s favorite activities before she got sick was mowing the lawn. I came home one afternoon to find D.D. in the front yard, covered with sweat, and the lawnmower running wide open. When I offered to take over for her, she took it to mean that I didn't think she was up to cutting the grass. She snapped, "What do you want me to do, lie in bed and die?" Enough said. That exchange made me keenly aware of how important it was for her to resume her normal pre-surgery activities as soon and to whatever extent possible.

Fortunately there was very little in D.D.'s former routine that she could not resume. We even resumed our pre-surgery sex life. It was great therapy for both of us, physically and emotionally.

The only adverse reaction D.D. encountered was pain in her back. She had suffered from a chronic back problem prior to her breast cancer diagnosis and initially dismissed its recurrence as being caused by excessive physical activity. But when the pain continued despite several days of rest, D.D. made an appointment to see John Carpenter. We both remembered all too well our procrastination in seeking medical advice about the nodule on D.D.'s breast. This time, if there was something wrong, we definitely wanted to know as early as possible.

After examining D.D., Dr. Carpenter told us that if her back pain was related to cancer, it was "old" cancer that had metastasized from her breast cancer. He explained that the massive amounts of chemotherapy she had taken before and after her operation made the existence of any new cancer very unlikely.

Always the thorough nurse, D.D. asked if he intended to send her for an MRI, which could resolve any doubt. Dr. Carpenter considered an MRI to be unnecessary, but D.D. was persistent and finally persuaded him to order the test. Call it a woman's instinct, a nurse's sixth sense, or whatever, D.D. apparently knew something because the MRI revealed lesions on her spine; a subsequent biopsy confirmed that they were malignant. Dr. Carpenter again told us that in his opinion the cancer was not new but had metastasized before D.D. began chemotherapy. I could not understand why, if that was the case, it hadn't shown up in an earlier test.

Even if it was "old" cancer, just knowing that D.D.'s cancer had metastasized sent us into a panic. We had great faith in Dr. Carpenter, but to calm our fears we decided to get a second opinion about the cancer in D.D.'s back.

We decided to go to M.D. Anderson Cancer Hospital in Houston for several reasons. I had heard about it for years and knew several people who had gone there for treatment, although none of them had breast cancer. It was a major cancer center and was much closer to us geographically than others, such as Sloan-Kettering in New York. We could get nonstop, reasonably priced air service to Houston, and Tina was there to provide ground transportation and a place to stay. When we told Tina about our decision to come to M.D. Anderson, she called and got us an appointment with Dr. Richard Theriault quicker than we could say "chemo-therapy."

When I saw the hospital complex in Houston I was really impressed by its size and the fact that every building and every staff member was devoted to treating nothing but cancer. The breast cancer clinic alone at M.D. Anderson took up more floor space than the entire oncology department we had gone to at Kirklin Clinic.

As usual I was as nervous as hell by the time we arrived at Dr. Theriault's office, but I calmed down after meeting him. He is a personable, warm, and engaging fellow and made us feel very comfortable. Like UAB's John Carpenter, Dr. Theriault is an expert in treating breast cancer, and we talked with him about everything—tamoxifen therapy, D.D.'s good general health, her operation, and most of all, the cancerous lesions that had shown up on her recent MRI. Dr. Theriault exuded confidence and gave us some general impressions from his review of D.D.'s records before he ordered a battery of tests, which we expected. We were greatly relieved that the results from the new tests were entirely consistent with those from Kirklin Clinic. Dr. Theriault told us that he concurred with Dr. Carpenter's assessment that tamoxifen should effectively control D.D.'s cancerous spinal lesions. He confirmed in direct terms what Dr. Carpenter had suggested more indirectly: The spinal lesions were not new cancer but had come from pre-mastectomy metastasis.

For continued peace of mind, we have decided to see both Dr. Theriault and Dr. Carpenter every three months to catch any recurring cancer as early as possible. We've shuttled back and forth to Houston a number of times now, and the routine is better than one might imagine. We go out one day for tests, and see Dr. Theriault before coming home the following day.

We continue to hope that the tamoxifen will keep D.D.'s cancer in remission.

It is very important to your wife that she resume her regular pre-surgery activities as soon as she can.

Remember that you have breast cancer, not had it. Be wary of every unexplainable symptom that indicates the cancer has recurred.

If you think you need a second medical opinion, get one. If you can't go across the country to get it, at least go across town.

READY TO EXPLODE

I have taken D.D.'s breast cancer as a personal assault on our lives, and to put it bluntly, it has pissed me off. I have taken an active stance and encouraged D.D. to pursue aggressive treatment—and I have physically and emotionally supported her every day since her diagnosis. But being on the sideline, so to speak, has caused a enormous buildup of anxiety and energy. Sometimes I have felt like I was ready to explode—I want to do something more to fight back against breast cancer.

Through the years I haven't felt that I have done anything to make much of a difference in the lives of other people, but in recent years I have felt the desire to do something that made an impact on other people's lives.

I was still chasing the vision of helping others when D.D. got sick. I have to admit that in this case my desire to help others was absolutely selfish: the "others" I focused on were D.D. and our son, Ben. I wanted to do something— raise money, anything—that would in some way extend D.D.'s life. Although I didn't think about helping anybody but D.D. and Ben, my idea for a charity golf tournament has come to fruition and raised almost $200,000 for breast cancer research in the past two years—money that hopefully will help not only D.D. but all breast cancer victims.

I'd known for a long time that golf tournaments annually raised millions of dollars for a myriad of charities. Some- where I heard that the Professional Golf Association gives more money to charities each year than the National Football

League, the National Basketball Association, and the National Hockey League combined. So a golf tournament was in the back of my mind, and the more I thought about it, the more I liked it. I especially liked the idea of a Ladies Professional Golf Association tournament: an event for women, involving women, to support women who needed help.

I shared my idea with my friend Louis Josof, a counselor at UAB's Comprehensive Cancer Center, and he suggested that I get in touch with Dolly O'Neal, who was an avid golfer as well as a breast cancer survivor. When I called Dolly, she agreed to meet with me. I decided to take along my friend and accountant, Norman Berk, whose wife is also a breast cancer survivor.

Our meeting was very successful. Although our interests in raising funds for breast cancer differed a little, we found a considerable amount of common ground and decided to join forces.

One of the first things we did was create a charitable non-profit corporation, The Breast Cancer Research Foundation of Alabama, to sponsor the golf tournament and make all decisions regarding the distribution of funds raised by the event. Norman had experience with charitable corporations, and his work in bringing the foundation to life was essential to our ultimate success. This part of the project, at least, went smoothly.

Otherwise the three of us were running around like the Keystone Kops. We were well into January and the LPGA could give us only one date, April 22, when its players might participate in our event. We had a mountain of work to do and less than four months in which to do it. We relied heavily on Larry Williams and others at UAB's Comprehensive Cancer Center for advice and assistance. Larry worked closely with us and introduced us to Charlie Baker, which led to a major breakthrough.

Fairly new to Birmingham, Charlie was an executive with Xerox Corporation and was interested in increasing Xerox's involvement with local charities in Birmingham, like the company had done in other cities. It didn't hurt that Charlie was also a golfer—he loved our idea for an LPGA tournament. He went to work right away, and Xerox became the principal sponsor of our event, which we named the "Xerox Drive Out Breast Cancer Golf Tournament."

We scheduled our tournament and brought in twenty-five LPGA professionals who were teamed with one hundred local players—not too shabby for our first time and with only four months to pull the whole thing together. The event turned out to be a great success, financially and otherwise.

I was delighted with our success, but even raising a lot of money didn't matter compared to what was really important—for D.D. to live a long, long time. I've reflected every day on how, even considering that we live in a time of incredible technological innovation, the human body has remained more complicated than all the computers, all the medicines, and all of the treatments combined. I'm constantly amazed that no cure for breast cancer has yet been found.

Of course the cure will come someday but I'm too selfish to be patient. Just thinking that D.D.'s metastatic cancer likely has shortened her life has made me even more impatient. I helped raise the money so some bright somebody could find a cure for her, not just for women in general. Once her cancer has returned, if it does, no matter how much money has been raised, it may not be enough. I believe D.D.'s destiny has been cast largely to luck and chance, neither of which has ever provided me much comfort or confidence.

I am truly terrified at the prospect of losing her. Tamoxifen has helped her a lot, but the doctors and statistics all indicate that the benefits will be good for about five years, and then she'll need something else. I'm afraid her luck will run out before "something else" is found.

Cheering from the sidelines while your wife does the actual fighting in your battle against breast cancer can cause an enormous buildup of anxiety and energy.

You may be mad enough to fight, but you won't be able to actually get your hands on the enemy. You will have to find another way to fight cancer.

IF IT'S NOT ONE THING, IT'S ANOTHER

Before D.D's mastectomy, we had serious, difficult choices to make about breast reconstruction. The simplest choice was having no reconstructive surgery, leaving just a scarred chest wall where her breast had been. It wasn't an option either of us considered for very long given D.D.'s relative youth and our desire for her to look as normal as possible.

The choices about what kind of reconstructive surgery to have were dramatically more difficult and involved. D.D. was a candidate for "immediate" reconstruction, meaning that Dr. Grotting would do the first of several reconstructive procedures as soon as Dr. Urist removed her breast during her Labor Day surgery. From the surgeon's point of view, immediate reconstruction has some technical advantages, including the skin flaps on the breast would be pliable and manageable. The primary benefit from our point of view was that D.D. would wake up from the mastectomy with a mound where her breast had been.

Another choice was to wait for D.D.'s mastectomy to heal, usually a minimum of three months, before starting the reconstruction process. Waiting would require a second major operation followed by one or more simpler procedures. All things considered, we decided D.D. would have immediate reconstruction, leaving only simpler procedures in which Dr. Grotting would later fashion a nipple on her reconstructed breast.

Next we had to decide what type of immediate reconstruction D.D. would have—which gave us additional difficult choices to make. Dr. Grotting explained that he could perform the reconstruction using either a saline implant or D.D.'s own body, which required lengthy major surgery to excise tissue from her abdomen and create a mound at the site of her mastectomy. Using D.D.'s own body tissue would make the reconstructed breast more natural than an artificial implant, which appealed to both of us. I especially wanted her "new" breast to be as natural and as much like the original as possible, and I was happy that she also wanted to use her own tissue. I was very naive about how the reconstruction would be done until I learned that Dr. Urist would remove all of the tissue from D.D.'s breast during the mastectomy. Then I could visualize just how much of her body would be needed to re-create her breast and why the surgery would be so long and tedious.

In the second reconstruction procedure, Dr. Grotting formed a nipple on the silver dollar-sized piece of skin that he had cut from D.D.'s abdomen and grafted into her "new" breast immediately after Dr. Urist completed her mastectomy. I was astonished and pleased by Dr. Grotting's attention to detail— he had chosen a portion of D.D.'s skin showing a small birthmark to ensure that the nipple would appear natural.

This second procedure was performed as outpatient surgery, and we arrived at the hospital at 7 a.m. for what was to be 9 a.m. surgery. After waiting all morning and through lunch, D.D. was finally taken to the operating room at 1:30 p.m. Dr. Grotting completed the procedure in less than an hour, and D.D. stayed in the recovery room for another hour or so before a nurse brought her into the small room where I was waiting. D.D. still felt lightheaded from the anesthesia and complained of nausea, but a nurse came in after what seemed to be just a few minutes and told me I could take D.D. home. When I questioned whether D.D. was ready to leave, the nurse gave me a vomit pan and said, "Once she gets home, she'll be all right."

It was 4:30 p.m. and D.D. was the last patient of the day— the sooner she went home, the sooner the nurse could leave. I was pissed off, but I decided not to argue with the nurse—I just wanted to get D.D. home as quickly as possible. I helped her into her loose-fitting clothing, noticed that her breast was again bandaged, eased her into a wheelchair, and pushed it toward the exit. D.D. threw up all the way to the car.

For the first time I saw in her face what I had heard and read about for months: how important a woman's breasts are to her sense of wholeness. In the long run she'd be glad to have gone through it, but her second surgery reminded her of losing her breast in the first place. No matter how long she might live, her beautiful body was gone forever. We both needed to grieve about that.

Life has also been an emotional roller coaster ride for us in ways not directly related to D.D.'s own surgery or treatment. We have met a lot of really nice people during our ordeal, folks who were going through their own cancer nightmares. Some of them are still alive and fighting, while others are not.

One of the people we came across was Susan, a young woman from Houston who Tina met at one of her support groups. D.D. had a great deal in common with Susan: Both of them were attractive, in their thirties, and had one child. Both had learned shortly after surgery that their cancers had metastasized to their spines. Both were patients of Dr. Theriault and were taking tamoxifen. Unfortunately tamoxifen had not worked for Susan and her cancer had recurred for a second time. She was preparing for a bone marrow transplant, a difficult and sometimes risky therapy. The news of Susan's misfortune demoralized D.D., not only because she liked Susan very much but also because they had so much in common. We both wondered whether D.D.'s favorable response to tamoxifen would last.

In May 1996, after D.D. had been taking tamoxifen for about four months, Dr. Robert Varner, her new gynecologist, discovered cysts on her ovaries. Fortunately test results proved they were benign, but it was a serious scare.

The presence of ovarian cysts prompted D.D. to become interested in Dr. Susan Love and her work in treating breast cancer. D.D.'s sister, Tina, had read Dr. Susan Love's Breast Book and her other books and had shared Dr. Love's theories with D.D. Dr. Love suggested that a premenopausal woman whose breast cancer had metastasized to her bone tissue should have her ovaries removed (an oophorectomy). Although I didn't grasp the medical details of this theory as well as D.D. and Tina did with their nursing background, I did understand that Dr. Love's ideas were the subject of some controversy within the medical community. Usually once D.D. makes up her mind about something, I don't try very hard to change it—and when D.D. decided to have an oophorectomy, I didn't say anything, at least not at first.

D.D. discussed the pros and cons of having an oophorectomy with Dr. Varner, who agreed to perform the procedure if she wanted it. He believed an oophorectomy would not hurt her and might help her, but he did not encourage her to go forward. When D.D. asked Dr. Carpenter and Dr. Theriault, about it, both of them said they could help D.D. without having her undergo any additional surgery, but neither of them discouraged her from having an oophorectomy. D.D. went ahead and set up a date for the procedure.

I had my own doubts about a thirty-six-year-old woman having an oophorectomy. My simplistic view is "If it ain't broke, don't fix it."

The more I thought about D.D. having an oophorectomy, the more angry I became. I resented the fact that she'd already had more surgery than anyone deserved, least of all her since she had done nothing to bring on her cancer. The whole thing was just so unfair. But D.D. insisted that having the oophorectomy was the right thing to do, so I went along with her.

We had an appointment to see Dr. Varner the day before the operation, which gave me an opportunity to meet him for the first time and hear firsthand about the surgery—what he would be doing and what we should expect as to hospitalization, recovery, and so forth. As I understood it Dr. Varner could perform the operation either vaginally or through D.D.'s abdomen, depending upon the accessibility of the ovaries. Each technique had its own recovery period.

Just being in Kirklin Clinic again brought back all of my feelings associated with D.D.'s diagnosis, chemotherapy, major surgery, and the outpatient surgery.

I listened closely as Dr. Varner explained the procedure. When we started asking him questions, I got the impression that he was not one hundred percent sure D.D. should undergo the operation. I relaxed a bit, but D.D. seemed miffed because she was all pumped up to go through with it. I mentioned the Susan Love theory to Dr. Varner, who explained that many doctors had a different opinion as to whether a woman in D.D.'s situation should have an oophorectomy. He said that he had found nothing in his examination of D.D. that required an oophorectomy. All of a sudden he seemed to be discouraging having the surgery, saying that he'd be watching D.D. closely enough that if an oophorectomy became necessary in the future, he'd schedule it then. I asked him what he would recommend if his wife was in D.D.'s situation. He replied that he would do everything he could to talk her out of having the surgery. Man, was I impressed! Having grown up hearing about surgeons being scalpel happy, here I was having a conversation with a doctor who did not want to operate.

I appreciated Dr. Varner's frankness and sincerity and felt relieved when D.D. agreed to cancel the operation. As D.D. and I drove home, however, she fretted that Dr. Carpenter might have talked Dr. Varner out of doing the surgery. I assured her that Dr. Varner had made his own decision based on his evaluation of her medical condition. But I also offered to go back to the clinic and reschedule the oophorectomy if she still wanted to have it. I was very relieved when she declined my offer.

By the time we got home I was emotionally frazzled. I left as soon as I could to go work out—something I have learned helps alleviate anxiety and frustration.

Just when you've finished weighing the options and making one difficult decision, you'll have to make another.

Write down questions as you think of them and keep asking your doctor until you get an answer— even though you may not want to hear the answer.

Exercise or do some other physical activity to help relieve the inevitable anxiety and frustration of fighting with cancer on a daily basis.

Keep your sense of humor. Try to find something to laugh about in every situation, no matter how bad it seems.

SEX, FEAR, AND INTENSIFIED EMOTIONS

Before D.D.'s diagnosis we had a mutually satisfying sex life, and I did not want to lose that vital part of our marriage. I worried a great deal about how chemotherapy, the mastectomy, and reconstruction surgery would affect us sexually. How would we deal with the physical changes in D.D.'s body? Would we feel too awkward or repulsed to openly enjoy physical intimacy? Would D.D.'s breasts still be a source of pleasure for both of us like they had been in the past?

We had never talked about sex before, other than to joke about it, but in the months since D.D.'s diagnosis we've had an ongoing dialogue about the differences in her body, which has helped us become even more intimate, sexually and otherwise. We made love regularly when she was bald, after her recovery from surgery, during the various stages of breast reconstruction, and in the midst of tamoxifen's menopausal-like side effects. And we've continued to enjoy sex even though we've found it to be different physically as well as emotionally. Making love means much, much more now, and it has a bittersweet edge. Before D.D.'s cancer I tended to take sex for granted, as a good thing that came with marriage. Now I just wonder how many more times we will be able to share that great coital mystery together. I cannot imagine being unable to hold and caress D.D.

I had heard stories about husbands who abandoned their wives after they were diagnosed with breast cancer, and I remembered one couple I had known many years earlier. The husband, a successful physician, had marched into the recovery room, where his wife was still reeling from anesthesia following her double mastectomy, and told her he wanted a divorce—and he got it. I couldn't understand then how he—or any other man—could abandon his wife, the mother of his children, in a time of crisis. But even though I have never considered abandoning D.D., I now understand how dealing with the stress, fear, and ugliness of breast cancer could make a husband want to run away from it all.

I realize that dealing with breast cancer has intensified my emotions. I suspect that if a couple has an intimate, loving relationship, cancer may bring them even closer together, like it has D.D. and me. On the other hand, if a couple has already drifted apart, dealing with cancer may end their relationship.

I continue to struggle to live one day at a time, to stay in the present without worrying about what the future may hold. I can't help myself, though—I worry about the future every day.

At the rational level I've accepted the fact that the fight against breast cancer is fraught with the uncertain, the inconclusive, and the unknown—but fear still rips at my gut. Sometimes I've worried so much that I fear I'll cause something else bad to happen to D.D., and I'm much more wary of bad news than D.D. is. Whenever she experiences the least little ache or pain, a twinge of terror runs down my spine.

Several months ago, for instance, D.D.'s thumb started hurting. She tried to live with the pain but finally went to the doctor, not only to relieve the discomfort but to get some peace of mind. All I could think about was the time I saw a friend who had to have part of his hand amputated because of recurrent cancer—and he died not long afterward. I was more than relieved when we found out the pain in D.D.'s thumb was only tendinitis.

I remember saying to Dr. Varner once that I'd come to realize that we'll never totally have peace of mind—there will always be something that causes us to agonize. He agreed, and told me that it was a natural reaction.

Before D.D.'s diagnosis, I worried that the difference in our ages meant that D.D. would be a relatively young woman when I died. Now the shoe is on the other foot.

Along with struggling to live one day at a time, I also struggle daily at home and work to worry only about those things I can do something about and let go of everything else, including the day, hopefully a long time from now, when we learn that D.D.'s cancer has recurred.

Dealing with breast cancer will intensify your emotions.

The stress, fear, and ugliness of breast cancer may make you want to run away from it all.

Having breast cancer means you'll never totally have peace of mind—there will always be something that will cause you to agonize.

Try to live one day at a time and to worry only about those things you can do something about. Let go of everything else, including the day, hopefully a long time from now, when your wife's cancer will recur.

I'M FOR
WHATEVER WORKS

I'm not a very religious person and I'm skeptical of praying for healing. Nevertheless I'm grateful for all the people who have been praying for D.D. and have placed her name on prayer lists.

I believe that there's a healing spirit within each of us, and it takes on different forms of expressions depending on what works for each individual. Some people believe religious practices are an integral part of healing. For others, including me, having a positive attitude is the key. I have chosen to believe that D.D. is strong enough to win her battle with cancer with my help and help from others.

D.D. grew up in the Roman Catholic faith, and prayers and religious practices are important to her. This summer she went with her family to Lourdes, France, to drink from the spring that, according to tradition, flows with healing holy water. She and I have floated in the Dead Sea and experienced the physical and spiritual uplifting of its salt waters. And we have rubbed our hands in "healing" dirt in New Mexico.

Basically, I'm for whatever works! And I know that whatever else we do—or anybody else does for us—we're going to need a lot more help from modern medicine to keep winning our battle with breast cancer.

Do whatever works for you, from keeping a positive attitude to following religious traditions.

FIGHTING THE HEALTH CARE SYSTEM AS WELL AS THE CANCER

We only recently received a substantial bill from Dr. Jim Grotting for the reconstructive surgery he performed some eighteen months earlier. We couldn't understand why the bill came so long after the operation until we found out that the doctor's office had submitted the bill earlier to our insurance company and our insurance company refused to pay it because the charge was "not reasonable and customary." We've heard that phrase—"not reasonable and customary"—at least a dozen times about charges for D.D.'s various treatments. Dealing with an insurance company can be almost as traumatic as dealing with breast cancer itself.

Sometimes I think insurance companies deal with people the same way they deal with cars—when you have an accident and make a claim, they tell you to get three estimates before they pay to have the damage fixed. When you have breast cancer, you don't want to have to go to three doctors and have the insurance company tell you to have the "damage" fixed by the doctor who gave the lowest estimate.

D.D. volunteered to be the go-between with our insurance company both because she was at home during business hours and had time to arm-wrestle with them. She thought her nurse's training might help her to understand why the company made a particular decision to pay or not to pay a claim. She found right off what most people learn, sooner or later—insurance companies do what they want to do. They put the burden squarely on the insured patient to prove what the company should pay. Many nights when I came home from work, D.D. would say in an exasperated tone, "Let me tell you what that stupid insurance company told me today."

We got rejection notices on bills months after the charges had been submitted. At least once the insurance company refused to pay a claim contending there had been double billing when, in fact, the insurance company had not processed the bill in a timely fashion and the doctor's office had merely resubmitted the original bill.

When we started having regular problems with our insurance company, I called the human resources department at my company's home office in Atlanta and talked with the person who handles the health insurance. "My wife has breast cancer," I told her. "We're fighting for her life—we don't need to be battling with the insurance company too. Can you make a call or two to help us out with this problem?" That got us some temporary relief at least.

I'd advise everyone to establish rapport with someone either in their company's personnel department or at their insurance company who can help with claims. Insurance companies may be faceless, conscienceless monoliths, but people, fortunately, are still human beings who tend to react more favorably and more efficiently when they know somebody, even if only over the telephone.

Dealing with hospital staffs and rules can be difficult too. I learned to ask lots of questions about what we could and couldn't do. I wanted to be by D.D.'s side for every test and treatment, and I made sure to ask every time, "Can I go in with her?" I even sat in on her MRI in Houston simply because we asked.

My biggest frustration with hospitals is the paperwork, paperwork, and more paperwork—primarily because doing all the paperwork involved giving the same information six or seven times. Every time we went to a different department in the same hospital, we had to answer the same questions. I wish hospitals would get their act together so patients could answer all the questions just once and the information would be available to all of the departments in the facility.

Crowded waiting rooms, lengthy delays, and sometimes impatient, insensitive, irritable receptionists and other support staff members added to D.D.'s and my stress. We wanted to focus all our time and energy on fighting the cancer, and instead we had to sit and wait and deal with sometimes overworked, seemingly insensitive staff members. We learned to take books or something else along with us to doctor's appointments and treatment sessions. About the only good thing about spending so much time in the clinics was talking with the nurses—many of them gave us very helpful, practical suggestions.

Occasionally we encountered problems that were more than merely annoying. For instance, sometimes all the nurses were on break when it was time to change the fluid during chemotherapy. The one thing that really made me mad was having someone at the hospital enter the wrong breast on D.D.'s surgery orders.

I once told one of our doctors that having a positive attitude and emotional strength is crucial to the healing process, but spending endless hours waiting for test results or to see a doctor was detrimental to one's mental and emotional well-being. He agreed—but that didn't make the waits any shorter.

I learned to accept all of these frustrations as just part of the health care system. I knew it wouldn't do any good by losing my cool and getting angry at the staff, so I took lots of deep breaths and tried to relax. It wasn't—and still isn't—easy, but I'm trying to work with the system rather than fighting it.

Dealing with your health insurance company can be almost as traumatic as dealing with breast cancer itself. Insurance companies sometimes seem to deal with people the same way they deal with cars—get three estimates and have the "damage" fixed by the cheapest bidder.

Establish rapport with someone either in your company's personnel department or at your insurance company who can help with claims. Fortunately insurance company employees are still human beings, and they tend to react more favorably and efficiently when they know you, even if only over the telephone.

Doctors agree that having a positive attitude and emotional stability enhances the healing process. Unfortunately the hours you spend waiting for test results or to see a doctor will wreak havoc with both your attitude and your emotions.

Seemingly inexcusable mistakes, the endless amount of paperwork, and the occasional somewhat rude behavior on the part of a hospital staff member will also wreak havoc with your emotional well-being.

Keep trying to work with the health care system rather than fighting it.

LOOKING BACK

No matter what I've done in life, there's a part of me that requires me to look back at what has transpired with an eye toward what I might have done differently, although not necessarily better. Given the life-changing events of dealing with breast cancer for over two years now, I've reflected on many things.

Every time I look at D.D.'s body, which is virtually every day, I am reminded of what she endured. She looks good, but sometimes I wish she looked the way she did before her mastectomy. Then there are her scars, the most remarkable of which is the massive one on her abdomen where flesh was taken to form a "new" breast. Months after the reconstruction surgery, D.D. told me that if she had to make the decision again, she'd opt to have a saline implant because her belly remains tight and sore unless she exercises every day. And she doesn't have much feeling around her "new" nipple— it's not sensitive like it used to be. I wonder what it would be like if we had made different choices.

Recently I ran into a friend who we used to see regularly at Kirklin Clinic with his wife, who was also in chemotherapy for breast cancer. He told me that he could not imagine how I continued to be involved with breast cancer. "When all of our operations and chemotherapy were over," he said, "I just needed to let it go and to put it behind me." My guess is that deep down he hasn't let go of it all. A husband's supportive role never really changes. How could it?

I check the obituary columns in the local papers almost every day now, something I never did until my friend and coworker Warren Merrin died three months after being diagnosed with cancer last year. I took Warren's death very personally, not only because of our friendship but because I realized how lucky D.D. and I are that she's still alive and doing well.

Every time I go jogging now, I think back to the running I did during the one-hundred-degree days in July and August 1995. I remember telling myself back then that if I could withstand the misery of the heat and humidity, I could handle anything else, meaning D.D.'s illness of course. She was suffering the ill effects of chemotherapy at the time, and I wonder if I was punishing myself physically by trying to even things out between us—I sometimes felt guilty that she was suffering and I wasn't. Or maybe I was simply trying to escape the inner pain I felt and didn't express openly.

You can't change the fact that your wife has breast cancer, but you can fight it with her by being with her as much as you can and telling her every day how much you love her.

Realize that you are going to feel angry, helpless, and inadequate because you can't control the disease. Let her know that you're hurting too.

Talk to someone about what you feel and are experiencing—it doesn't matter whether it's a therapist, a support group, or just your best friend, talk it out.

When you feel that you're about to go over the edge emotionally, talk with a doctor; if you don't have your own doctor, talk with your wife's doctor.

Take an occasional sleeping pill, prescribed antidepressant medication, or whatever you need to do to keep yourself strong—so you can continue to provide strong support for your wife.

Take care of yourself physically too—get regular checkups, eat right, exercise, and get enough rest.

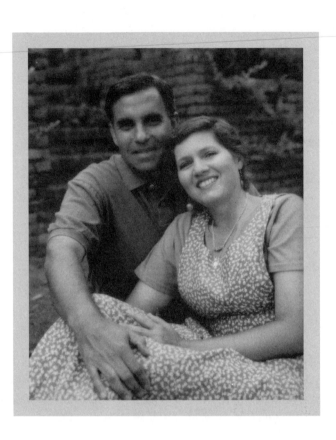

WAITING

Dr. Carpenter once told us, "When the cancer recurs, we'll know more." I immediately asked, "Don't you mean to say *if*, not *when?*" He answered, with a tone of conviction in his voice, "No, it will recur."

That was a difficult and painful statement for me to hear—D.D. has breast cancer, not had it. Her cancer is in remission, tamoxifen seems to be working—but the cancer may become active again, nobody knows when. Although D.D.'s tests, both in Birmingham and Houston, continue to be favorable, her cancer remains in her back.

We're stuck in a waiting game—a deadly waiting game.

D.D. looks great and feels good, but there are daily reminders of the truth: Her hair and skin are different (her skin is actually more beautiful) as the result of chemotherapy. Tamoxifen has caused premature menopausal symptoms. Her navel was moved four inches and her belly is still uncomfortably tight as the result of reconstructive surgery. Her back still hurts, although not so much as before. She has scars all over her body.

D.D. is incredibly tough and tenacious. She will fight for her life with everything she has within her. If breast cancer beats her, it will have to win what surely will be the mother of all battles. I know D.D. will fight fiercely; I can only hope that her cancer will throw in the towel, tuck tail, and run.

But I have to be realistic. If she loses the battle, I want her to die with dignity and with the knowledge that she missed out on very little in life. For that reason we stay busy, without making a big deal of it. How ironic it is that we're having the best years of our lives together at the same time I'm struggling with the uncertainty of the future.

Despite my reluctance to ask questions about D.D.'s long-term prognosis, I once asked Dr. Theriault how long a person with cancer metastasized to the bone could expect to live. He said the longest he ever heard of was forty-two years. I told him we intended to break that record.

> *Dealing with breast cancer is like being stuck in a waiting game—a deadly waiting game.*

CANCER MAY BE KILLING D.D., BUT IT'S NOT KEEPING HER FROM LIVING

Four days after I reviewed the final manuscript for this book, I got a telephone call from D.D., who was in Frankfurt, Germany, on a trip with her family. She told me that she'd just gotten word that Dr. Theriault wanted her to stay over in Houston on her way home to Birmingham to have a CAT scan to clear up a suspicious MRI result. D.D. had an MRI done at M.D. Anderson right before she left on her trip, and the results indicated a recurrence of her metastatic cancer that, by all previous accounts, had been in remission.

When I hung up the telephone, I immediately called Dr. Theriault to find out more about the test results. Personable as always, Dr. Theriault said that he was sorry to have to tell me that it looked like the tamoxifen was no longer effective.

I had remained upbeat the whole time I worked on this book. D.D. looked good, felt good, and her tests results were good. I was sure she was getting well. During the editing process I lobbied my coauthor and editor to deemphasize that the doctors had told us that D.D.'s cancer will return. I was more comfortable with words like may, possibly, or conceivably. They sounded better to me not only because they were less certain but because they described what I believed, that D.D. was going to beat breast cancer. The doctors were just being cautious. They only needed to look at D.D. to see how healthy she was.

Then without warning, a single telephone call gave me an unwelcome but much-needed shot of reality. For the first time I grasped the difference between believing what I desperately wanted to believe, that D.D.'s cancer was gone forever, and the numbing truth, that her cancer had recurred. I had fallen into the same trap that catches so many others—I was in denial.

Not only had I denied Dr. Carpenter's counsel that D.D.'s cancer would return, I had downright ignored it. I believed—because I wanted to believe—that everything was going to work out fine for D.D. and me. Tamoxifen would carry us for five years or more, and it would be at least that long before we had to face any more bad news. I had not prepared myself for this circumstance, and I was not ready when it came. I wondered whether I would ever be ready for bad news.

I felt angry and frightened all over again, just as on the first day D.D. told me she had breast cancer. I felt very much alone. In fact, I was alone; D.D. and Ben would not be home from their trip for another twenty-four hours. I tried to get my mind off the subject by reading and watching television, but I found myself over and over on the telephone, sharing the bad news with family and friends, almost anyone who would listen. I worried about how D.D. was handling the discovery, but I realized that she had her family with her.

I had no one with me, and I missed D.D. terribly. I was thrilled and relieved to see her and Ben when they stepped off the airplane Friday evening. It had been a long seventeen days.

Dr. Carpenter was neither surprised nor alarmed by the recurrence of D.D.'s cancer. It was what he'd expected all along.

Estrogen was the most likely culprit for the cancer's return; tamoxifen had not controlled the effects of her body's estrogen enough to stifle her potent, aggressive cancer. Dr. Carpenter started D.D. on Zoladex, a drug that is injected into the body every three months. We hope it will shut down the production of estrogen by her ovaries and thus retard the growth of her cancer.

We learned that because the cancer was not going away and since it had not metastasized to a major organ where its development would be more rapid, stopping the production of estrogen provided D.D. the best chance for controlling her cancer's growth. Dr. Carpenter assured us that his recommended treatment was right where we wanted to be. Dr. Theriault agreed, in a later telephone conference with D.D.

We have survived another scare. There will be others, some undoubtedly more serious.

I know now that I will have to deal with more bad news, and I don't relish the thought of doing so. Dr. Carpenter told us that there's no new "miracle drug" coming down the pipeline to cure D.D. I told him that D.D had tasted holy water in Lourdes, floated in the Dead Sea, and rubbed her hands in healing dirt in Chimayo, New Mexico. I also told him that I did not believe any of it would heal her, but that I did believe in D.D.'s extraordinary strength and fortitude. He answered that I should have faith in whatever works for me. I also told him that if he would continue to do his job, we will continue to do ours—we will not give up.

The fact is, breast cancer may be killing D.D., but it's not keeping her from living.

Prepare yourself for the inevitable bad test results that will come someday—you will feel angry and frightened all over again.

No matter what, don't give up—keep on fighting.

Most of all, keep on living.

Afterword

by Deidre Bergeron Sokol

When Bruce started talking about writing a book about breast cancer, I wasn't sure what to think. I could not believe that he was really going to tell the world about all of the things we went through. Most of all, though, I could not believe that anybody else would be interested in my—our—experience.

Then as the book started to come together and as I read several of the drafts, I began to change my mind. Seeing our story written down in black and white was pretty interesting after all. It was scary, too, to look back at some of the hardest times. Ours was not terribly different from the ordeals of other couples we have gotten to know. It occurred to me that the book might enrich the situations of not only husbands, families, and friends, but of cancer patients themselves. Bruce's words also touch those of us who have or have had breast cancer by enhancing our understanding of what our significant others may feel as they battle the disease with us.

When Bruce wrote that we'd become emotionally closer after I was diagnosed with breast cancer, he was right. After he and I got back together following our separation we were closer in some ways, but we continued to drift along, so to speak. Without the intervention of some force to bond us together, we might have continued to drift apart, perhaps for good. But not now—no way it will happen.

I have heard the horror stories about men deserting their wives when breast cancer came calling, but I'm happy to say that I do not know one woman to whom that happened. And for Bruce and me, exactly the opposite was true—after my diagnosis our marriage became stronger than ever, in almost every way I can imagine. I frankly believe that God gave me breast cancer knowing that Bruce would do something for himself, for me, and for us. Except for having the cancer, which I'd gladly give back to God in the blink of an eye, of course, things couldn't have worked out better for Bruce and me—and for Ben too. Bruce has been marvelously supportive of me—more attentive, more available, more focused on our relationship and on his relationship with Ben—since that horrible day back in 1995 when I received the news that I have cancer. We really do love each other, absolutely unconditionally.

I'm proud of the way Bruce and I have hung in there with each other, and proud of him for all of the things he has done to try to help other people with breast cancer and the people who love those people. The golf tournament and this book are the main things, but I've learned over the past two years that Bruce really cares about other people and their problems. He can't "fix" cancer, but that doesn't deter him from trying.

As for myself, I'm feeling very strong these days, not that I have any illusions about invincibility. But I exercise regularly. I can run hard for nearly an hour. I have returned to working in my yard, which I love. As with everybody in my predicament, what comes next, comes when it comes. But not knowing what tomorrow may bring makes living life one day at a time a little bit easier.

Birmingham, Alabama
August 1997